Dr. David's
FIRST HEALTH BOOK OF
MORE
(NOT LESS)

MORE food,
MORE sex,
MORE faith
and everything else you
need for health,
happiness and
longevity.

DR. DAVID LIPSCHITZ
CO-AUTHOR RILEY LIPSCHITZ

BIOGRAPHY

David Lipschitz, MD, a world expert on longevity directs the Longevity Center at St. Vincent Medical Center after retiring as Chairman of the Donald W. Reynolds Department of Geriatrics and Institute on Aging at the University of Arkansas for Medical Sciences, a program ranked in the top 10 by US News and World Report, He is consistently recognized as "one of the best doctors in America"

Affectionately known as Dr. David, he has appeared on the Today show and CBS Sunday morning with Charles Osgood. He is featured weekly on Little Rock's NBC affiliate, KARK and has a live weekly medical radio show on KARN news radio called "ReCenter Your Life.

An article entitled "Doctors Wisdom Comes with Age" recently appeared on the front page of the Dallas Morning News. He has a nationally syndicated column "Life Long Health", a 26-part award-winning program on the PBS network entitled "Aging Successfully with Dr. David" and has written BREAKING THE RULES OF AGING, a popular book in which he dispels the myths of aging. He is a beloved physician who truly listens to his patients and even in the very old can miraculously improve and save lives. More importantly his goal is not to prolong life but assure that the life you have is of the highest possible quality.

In his 60's and nowhere near his prime, Dr. David will tell you – the best is yet to come.

Dr. David's FIRST HEALTH BOOK OF MORE (NOT LESS)

ACKNOWLEDGEMENT

My thanks to my daughter Riley who helped with every aspect of writing this book. No father could be more proud of you. A brilliant, wise beyond her years, young woman who is about to enter medical school. Your future cannot be more bright.

To my family, my harshest and most constructive critics, who keep me centered and honest. I love you all.

Thanks to my friends and colleagues at the University of Arkansas for Medical Sciences for supporting and standing behind me for over 30 years. No medical school in the nation has made a greater commitment to the research, education and to the care of older persons.

My thanks to Fred Smith, Steve Anderson and the board of the Donald W. Reynolds Foundation. Their support created the Donald W. Reynolds Department of Geriatrics and Institute on Aging that I headed until July 2008. Because of the foundation, this program is far and away the best of its kind in the nation and has consistently ranked in the top 10 as a postgraduate program by US News and World Report.

Thanks to Peter Banko, his colleagues and the board of St. Vincent Infirmary Medical Center in Little Rock as well as the leadership for the Catholic Health Initiative for their confidence in me and establishing the Longevity Center. The goal of providing affordable, accessible and rational care for the baby boomers and their parents has the potential of developing a model that has the potential of revolutionizing the way we deliver health care.

And last but not least as a native South African and a naturalized citizen my love for the State of Arkansas and the United States of America runs deep. Sadly too many of us take the advantages of being an American for granted. What a privilege to be part of this great country that has provided me with freedoms and possibilities beyond my wildest dreams.

DEDICATION

I dedicate this book to the thousands of patients, most of whom are over the age of 65 that I have cared for and come to know so well. They are sages and mentors who have influenced me greatly. From them I have learned what it takes to live a long and independent life. Their experiences have molded my thoughts and led me to develop the plan described in this book.

To my late father Henry who influenced me greatly and to my mother Hanid, my hero, who has embraced life to the fullest and at age 86 remains full of vim and vigor a shining example of a passionate life lived to the fullest.

To Alexa and the late William Dillard, whom I love as if they were my own parents. I have learned so much from you including the importance of hard work, honesty, commitment and the true meaning of success.

To Regina Goodhart and Frank and Dorothy Robbins who more than anyone taught me the importance of hope and faith in dealing with adversity and living a truly good life.

To Patricia and the late Willard Walker and their family who are shining examples of humanity at its best. Their charity comes with an inspiring humility and gratitude at the opportunity of being be able to give back so much to those in need.

To Melinda K Hall a woman I have never personally met. Her brilliant and humorous art has inspired me greatly and helped me recognize the powerful role that creativity in any form plays in making a life richer.

CHAPTER I INTRODUCTION
THE KEY TO HEALTH IS MORE – NOT LESS

Americans are fortunate to have the unalienable rights to life, liberty, and the pursuit of happiness. At our very core, the essence of being an American is to get the most out of life – the _continued_ pursuit of more happiness, more joy, and more freedom. And yet, when it comes to health, it's just LESS, LESS, LESS. Less food, less fat, less risk, less freedom!

Unfortunately, when it comes to longevity, the wisdom teaching deprivation and "less is more" is just plain WRONG. I have been helping patients navigate old age for the last 30 years – and, trust me, the people who live the longest, healthiest, and happiest lives seek MORE – not less. More sex, more love, more faith, more exercise, and even more food! For my most successful patients, life is about squeezing every morsel of happiness and joy from every minute of every day.

My patients come in all shapes and sizes – thick and thin, tall and short. Believe me, the exterior image of health is only the tip of the iceburg. Usually, that exterior image never really reveals the truth about health – or longevity. Thin doesn't mean healthy. Fat doesn't mean unhealthy. In our image-obsessed culture, we've lost sight of what it means to be _healthy_ rather than _look_ healthy.

The key to lifelong health is not about how you look – but rather how you live. Are you happy? Are you passionate? Do you love life?

Pursuing Happiness After 50

Though we likely give it little thought, we live in the only nation in the world that places happiness at the very core of its existence. At every age and every stage of life, we seek to be happy. But ever since the founders of this country wrote of our right to _pursue happiness_, generations of Americans have been asking the same question: "What does it take to be happy?"

Is happiness found in our work? In the things we acquire? In our relationships? our cars? our money? our children? our parents?

An interesting thing happens with age: the answer changes. What it means to be happy at age 25 is distinctly different than at 45 and it changes again by age 80. With age, the pursuit of happiness sheds a different light. The material things become less fulfilling. The accolades at work may seem less satisfying and the fancy car less important. The things that once fueled the very source of our happiness become less and less important. Once you realize that you have more years behind you than ahead, life changes!

In over 30 years of practicing medicine, this has been my greatest lesson: aging is a unique journey that will change you. People tend to think about the aging process only in a physical or medical way. Yes, your body will change, but the physical changes are only the tip of the iceberg when it comes to navigating this journey. You will grow and evolve. Your relationships will change. Your outlook on life will change—and your beliefs will change as well.

During my time as a geriatrician, I've had the privilege of helping thousands of patients journey through old age. The journey is different for each patient. Some age well while others age poorly. Some face illness with tenacity and vigor while others lose hope and give up. Some remain fit and agile while others dwindle away before my eyes. And for every one of those extremes, there are thousands of adults in the middle who navigate aging with peaks and valleys, ups and downs.

Every patient who walks through my door teaches me something about health and aging. Our relationship goes both ways—I help them promote health and prevent disease, and they help me understand the unique process of growing older.

My own journey

I wrote my first book, *Breaking the Rules of Aging,* in 2001, and in it I outlined what I believed to be the basics of longevity: *health* and *happiness*. When the book was published, I was 58 years old—a spring chicken, compared to most of my patients!

Much has happened since *Breaking the Rules of Aging. My* youngest son is now a junior in college and my eldest two sons have became fathers. For the first time in 26 years, my wife and I are living alone: official empty-nesters! Today I manage two chronic diseases and my wife has two as well. Last year I received my Medicare card and this year my first social security check.

The geriatrician has become geriatric.

Facing all these changes—the empty nest, being a grandfather, my own health challenges—I began to grapple with the same questions and concerns that every 65-year-old must face. Would I retire? What would I do? How can I be a good grandparent when I live 1000 miles away? How will my wife and I handle living alone? What was my purpose in life *today*? Eating healthy food and exercising seemed miniscule in the shadow of these larger *health* questions.

As I embarked on my own journey of navigating life in the Medicare era, I found myself looking back to those special patients who truly changed the way I viewed aging. These were the people that I looked up to and emulated. They approached each day with passion, vigor, and a zest for life. For them, neither money, nor fame, nor success stood in for the true happiness they felt from within. They are engaged human beings who live each year, month, day, and hour as if it were precious. They never felt "over the hill" or "past their prime"—in fact, they act as if every day is an opportunity to do more, give more, and be better.

Honestly, these inspiring patients were the very source of my prescription for lifelong health. They provided the model for the rest of us to follow! They took care of themselves, embraced their faith, exuded love and confidence, and remained engaged until the very end. They never retired from life.

But now that I found myself in the ranks of "geriatrics," I saw these patients in a new light. They had more than just health and happiness. They had that "it" factor that made them special and unique. With a little reflection, I realized that what they had was an enthusiasm about life that made them able to assure longevity. They were passionate about everything in life. No matter what it was—family and friends, successes and failures, illness and health—these people chose to pursue life to the fullest. They withdrew all worries, fears, and expectations and simply followed the path of passion.

For me to pursue happiness in this "third age" of life, it was clear that I too needed this enthusiasm and passion to achieve longevity. In the business of work, family, and everyday life, passion somehow got lost in the shuffle. Before I knew it, 65 was upon me and life has flown by. After 26 years of raising my children and building a career, I needed a renewed for passion for my work, my family, and my life.

This realization has major consequences. Ultimately, what we all must ask ourselves is this: why am I doing this if I don't *love* it? Whatever "it" is—from work to relationships—renewing passion in your daily life is the key to longevity. My patients paved the way for *me* to live life to fullest, because they had passion. Passion infused everything they do—and, every day, I aspire to have that same passion.

Finding passion in every element of your life is the magic bullet that increases the chances of longevity but more importantly to a better, healthier, and happier existence. Be passionate about your relationships. Be passionate about your family. Be passionate about your health and take care of your body. Be passionate about your career or your avocation. We have so little time on this earth; why waste it with mediocrity?

So here I was at 66 at the height of my career, widely accepted as a highly successful academician having built a world renowned aging institute that has received wide spread recognition. The Donald W. Reynolds Institute on Aging that I headed is ranked in the top 10 by US News and World Report an incredible success story. But at age 65 I believed new blood was needed to move this program to the next level. I stepped down and have taken on a new challenge – Director of the Longevity Center at St. Vincent a large community hospital that lies a short distance from the medical school. Now I have a new passion, I work harder than ever, I am nowhere near the prime of life and just love what I am doing.

Passion means laying it all on the line at any age. If you do that, you can't help being happy—and healthy.

Why me?

I am not your typical physician. The "typical" physician lives in a box with very clear boundaries. Each new patient is an opportunity to find a new disease, prescribe a new medication, and cure a new condition. This type of physician lives solely to fix problems. I don't. As a geriatrician, fixing problems is only one small piece of the health puzzle. For the last 25 years, I have been learning to approach health in a way that doesn't necessary "save" lives, but rather improves them.

For the majority of my career, I have been somewhat of a medical entrepreneur—not the kind who builds new businesses, but rather the kind who bucks the trend and finds new ways to grow and improve. Rather than sticking to one medical specialty, my path twisted and turned, touching on research, clinical care, teaching, and administration. From my initial training as a medical student, to academic research on aging, to the last ten years of running the nation's largest and most successful geriatric program, all of my experiences in medicine have culminated in a "perfect storm" that has truly prepared me to change the way Americans age.

Let's start at the beginning. I studied medicine at one of the most outstanding medical schools in the world, the University of the Witwatersrand in Johannesburg, South Africa, and received my MD in 1966. The training I received was unique because we were taught to be *bedside* physicians first. We were trained to be intellectual physicians who used our brains rather than relying on a huge battery of tests. My greatest mentor and teacher, Dr. Harry Seftel, frequently said, "Any fool can examine a patient, but it takes a genius truly to understand the person you evaluate, every aspect of their lives, as well as their medical problems." Believe me, this is the long-lost technique of *listening* to your patients and intuiting what's wrong. We were taught that everything could be learned through a medical history and evaluation. The blood tests were meant to be the back-up confirmation of an initial diagnosis. Being thoughtful and rational were the keys to medical success. Granted, this was in 1960s—well before the medical and technological advances commonplace today. Ultimately, I was taught to be a physician who could strip away the trappings of "modern medicine" and evaluate any patient from a comprehensive perspective.

Though I did not know it at the time, this training laid the groundwork for my career as a geriatrician. That emphasis on bedside manner and treating patients as people fuels my everyday work with older adults. What's more, it's the basis for this book. The older we get, the more complex our clinical problems become. New chronic conditions pile on with each passing decade, so it's imperative that every physician understand the comprehensive nature of health. The more experience you have, and the more careful you are, the more likely you will be able to make an accurate diagnosis and come up with the appropriate treatment plan.

Though I had a strong background in clinical care, I spent most of my early medical career in research. I worked with the world's leading authorities on hematology and iron metabolism, Dr. Thomas Bothwell in South Africa and Dr. Clement Finch from Seattle, Washington. After earning my Ph.D under Dr. Bothwell, I immigrated to the United States and had the incredible privilege of working under the direction of Dr. Finch, a true pioneer and one of the greatest physicians of the twentieth century. During that time, I developed a unique expertise, learning everything about the blood system. Research is about seeking—seeking new ideas, new thoughts, and new ways of approaching the traditional paradigm. My research in blood overlapped with many other medical fields, including oncology, nutrition, and geriatrics. After moving to the University of Arkansas for Medical Sciences in Little Rock, I dove into research on the effects of growing older on the bone marrow. Looking at anemia and aging, I developed a deep understand of what happens to the body with age. Ultimately, this opened the door to the totally new and emerging field of geriatrics.

While at the University of Arkansas, I had the good fortune of working at the Little Rock Veterans Administration Hospital with Dr. Eugene Towbin, one of the first pioneers of geriatrics (the clinical care of older persons) and gerontology (the study of the aging process). He told me that if I wanted to study the aging process, I should spend time taking care of older persons. That advice and urging changed my life forever.

There I was, a researcher thrown out of the lab and back to the clinic. At first, I didn't "get it." Geriatrics was a very young field and most primary care physicians did not believe fully in its value. What's more, I was so intently focused on the research that it took me a moment to see beyond it. After a while, I began to understand that an aging body—as well as an aging person—has unique health needs. A successful geriatrician relies on a completely different paradigm of medicine, one that looks at the patient as a whole rather than any single disease or problem. I also found that geriatrics was much more expansive than I ever imagined. Just as it takes a village to raise a child, it takes a village to care for an older adult. Our success relied on cultivating that village of healthcare experts, from physicians and nurses to social workers and pharmacists, dietitians, and rehabilitation experts. Learning to be a geriatrician called on every resource I had: the bedside training in Johannesburg and my research, as well as every sage word of advice I'd received from my many mentors along the way. I realized that this was my calling, that *thing* that I was meant to do.

Ever since then, I have been passionate about my craft. No longer a hematologist or internist, I now refer to myself as a *born-again geriatrician,* evangelical about the unique needs of an aging adult.

For the past 20 years I have had the privilege of taking care of thousands of older adults. During that time, I have learned a great deal, not just about aging, but about health as whole and navigating the health system at any age. This book is a combination of all these lessons – each step the product of my experiences, observations, and research. But, most of all, this book is about my own search for a passionate life. It's a tribute to all of my patients who taught me every lesson on living life well.

Your age is just a number

Your age is just a number. How *well* you age is completely up to you.

The aging process is best defined as *a complex interaction between an individual with his or her environment over time.*

There are three basic elements to aging: you, your environment, and time. These are the keys to how you age, how young you feel, and when illnesses develop.

- **You (and those before you).** You are a unique human being with a unique genetic makeup. The sad fact of aging is that some of it is left up to chance. Do you have good genes? Does longevity run in the family? If you have parents and relatives who remained healthy and happy well into their 90s, your chances of being like them are much higher than if your parents died at a younger age. These longevity genes determine your susceptibility to illnesses such as heart disease, diabetes and cancer.

- **Your environment.** This is far more important than the health of your parents or any longevity gene. How healthy you are after 60 greatly depends of factors *you* control. How well do you treat your body? Do you exercise? Are you stressed? Do you eat well? Did you develop healthy habits early in life? Were you exposed to pollutants in your environment? Your lifestyle and the environment you create play huge roles in how well you age.

- **Time.** Sooner or later, time will take its toll. We are all mortal and, ultimately, time wins. With each passing decade, your risk for developing diseases grows exponentially. By the age of 65, twenty percent of the population has memory loss. By age of 85, 50% of the population is physically or mentally dependent. These problems are not due to age, but rather illnesses that may be preventable. For the "oldest old"—individuals age 85 and up— time is not on their side. But the goal is not to lengthen one's time, but rather to improve the quality of each day.

All three of these factors combine to make you who you are, whether you're 35, 55, or 95. You cannot control time and you cannot control you genetic makeup, but you *can* control your environment, your lifestyle, and your attitude toward health. You may be predisposed to diabetes or have naturally high cholesterol. If you ignore it, don't take care of yourself, and do all the wrong things, you will develop chronic illnesses. If you develop illness later in life, your age certainly doesn't help you out.

Let me set the record straight: disease is not a function of aging. The effect of age on the brain, heart, lungs, and every other organ system is essentially inconsequential. Ultimately, the main effect of aging is a loss of resilience and reserve. This simply means that when stressed by an illness or exertion, an older body does not respond as rapidly or as well as a younger body. This loss of reserve makes the impact of an illness more severe and has greater consequences. So, as we grow older, we are more likely to develop an illness, our ability to respond to illness decreases, and the risk of complications may increase. Aging is a natural, biological process, but not the culprit for feeling "older." Disease and illness make us look, feel, and act old!

What we commonly think as "age-related" illnesses don't have to be age-related! The key is prevention. Prevent diseases or illnesses from occurring in the first place, and your age is simply a number.

A call to baby boomers: start now!

If you are healthy today, my message is even more crucial. **Do not wait** to start living the kind of life that promotes health, prevents disease, and ensures happiness. Living a healthy life after 60 is about *everything*—your food, your fitness, your stress, your family, your relationships, your sex, your faith, your passion. It's time to stop thinking about health simply in the context of your physical well-being. At 85, who cares if you have a bum leg or high cholesterol when you're unhappy, unloved, and sexless? The key to being healthy at any age is tapping in to your own passion for life. Surround yourself with love and greet each moment with a light-hearted smile. Stop stressing about everything and learn to enjoy yourself! This is the best insurance policy you'll ever buy.

If you're a baby boomer, consider yourself part of a long continuum—from the youngest of your generation to the oldest. In 2007, the first baby boomer signed up to receive Social Security, and that's the start of the scale. As each one of you turns a year older, the scale tips further, and more and more Americans will feel the impact of an aging nation.

If you want to ward off the effects of an aging body, mind, and spirit, this book is for you. The younger you are, the more important. It's never too early or too late to take care of your health, but the earlier your start the better. At age 60, your life expectancy is close to 30 years. At age 70, it's 16 years; at 80, it's 10 years; and at 90, it's six years. That's a long time! Take a lesson from the words of the great composer Eubie Blake: "If I'd known I was going to live this long, I would have taken better care of myself!" You have many, many years ahead of you. How do you want to live them?

It's in this context of helping Baby Boomers gear up for a new phase of life and love that I developed **Dr. David's Longevity plan**—10 things that we all need to do *more* of to find long lasting health and happiness.

Step 1. More passion. After age 50, nothing is worth doing if you don't really care about it. Feeling negative or neutral about any aspect of your life just simply isn't worth it! If you don't love your work, your relationships, where you live, what you eat—do something about it. Heed the words of Maya Angelou: "If you don't like something, change it. If you can't change it, change your attitude." Your time is precious, so be passionate about it. Get involved and excited about every aspect of every minute of your life.

Step 2. More peace and less stress. We stress about everything today, especially our health. It's time to stop stressing and find a little peace in life. Stress is the single most important factor leading to disease. Most importantly, it hinders us from doing all the other things necessary to live a healthy life. Learning to cope with stress must be a very high priority. This is not easy to do; it's a skill to be learned.

Step 3. More love. For many of us, love after 65 is a whole new world. But the more you love, the longer you live. Men who maintain long-standing, loving, monogamous and intimate relationships live an additional 10 years over single men! As marriages evolve and spouses face new challenges in life, it's even more important to take stock of your relationship and evaluate areas for improvement. Remember, love comes in many forms, from the intimate love between spouses to a community of love between friends, family, and neighbors. Infuse more love in your life and you'll be well on your way to a healthier tomorrow.

Step 4. More (and better) sex. Who doesn't want better sex? It's not a major predictor of longevity, but it's certainly fun to be passionate about! If you and your spouse want to pursue a more sexual relationship, there are plenty of ways to do it. Believe me, sex in the Medicare era can be more complete and satisfying than it was when we were younger.

Step 5. More faith and more prayer. It should come as no surprise that more faith is a key element of health after 65. As we age, it seems part of the natural progression to become more interested in faith and spirituality. There is compelling evidence linking faith and health. Those who believe in higher power live longer and respond to illness better than those that who don't. It's not what faith you belong to, or whether you attend religious services, but rather your *spirituality* that impacts health. If you are a good, loving, giving and—most importantly—*for*giving person, you will be a healthier person as well.

Step 6. More self-love. As a nation (and a generation) it's time we start loving ourselves more. Feeling good about yourself and comfortable in your own skin is a powerful predictor of longevity. Self-love is similar to self-esteem, but more expansive and encompassing. You may not identify with having low self-esteem, but we have all had periods without self-love. Loving yourself is the first step to loving others and it will open the door to a world of peace and contentment.

Step 7. More food. It's definitely time to restore our passion for food! We've become so obsessed with weight, pounds, and pants size, that most Americans have a totally unhealthy relationship with food. Diets fail: you never lose as much weight as you want, and, if you do lose weight, it typically comes right back. Our unhealthy obsession with thinness keeps us unhappy, disheartened, and frustrated. From a longevity perspective, a few extra pounds actually confer a survival advantage! That's right: the chubby among us actually live longer than those who are below their "ideal weight." Food is not the enemy. In fact, good food fuels your body and keeps you healthier longer. This step is not a black-and-white prescription of what you should and should not eat. Rather, it's about helping you cultivate a healthier relationship with food and educating yourself about the facts of healthy nutrition.

Step 8. More exercise. If there is one longevity pill that will improve the quality of your life, give you energy and enthusiasm, and prevent illnesses, it's exercise. Resistance training and aerobic exercise are essential components of living a healthy life. The more you exercise the better. But you don't have to go overboard and be crazy about it! Get out and walk—briskly—as much as you can. Even walking two hours a week has been shown to reduce your risk of heart disease by 40%.

Step 9. More empowerment to navigate the health system. The American health system is dysfunctional and not prepared for the aging of America. The United States ranks last in longevity when compared to every other developed country. American health care is so focused on high technology and acute care that the boring work of disease prevention is thrown to the wayside. What's more, health care is so profit-driven that when you do get sick, your physician will likely conduct the most aggressive tests, prescribe the most expensive drugs, and send you home with little more than a pat on the back and a thinner wallet.

Despite all this, you cannot avoid the health care system altogether. In order to ensure your own health and longevity, it's crucial to be impassioned about your own medical care. You have got to learn to *navigate* the system. You must engage with the health system early in order to detect and prevent disease. **Most importantly, you must be an empowered and educated consumer of health care.** You need to know the who, what, when, where, and why of every medical encounter. Who should you see? When should you go to the doctor? Where should you go? What can you expect? Why is a test conducted? Be personally involved in every health care decision and **never blindly believe everything your doctor tells you.** Physicians are human, have biases, and are under pressures of time and money. The decisions we make may by wrong. Seek second opinions and, if a treatment is prescribed, ask the critical questions. Why is this being recommended? Will it cure me? Will it prolong my life? Will it relieve symptoms and improve my quality of life? What are the side effects? The more serious the problem, the more critical these questions become.

Step 10. More freedom. At 66, I don't fit into any prepared box of what I'm supposed to do or where I'm supposed to be. For me, a big part of being healthy is being free to break the mold of what it means to be geriatric! For the last 40 years, baby boomers have been pushing the boundaries of American culture; why would we stop now? This final step is about pulling it all together and breaking all the rules. Be free to live where you want. Be free to work until the end. Be free to start a new life altogether. Be free to run for office or give back to the community. Be free to buck the trends and stop dieting. Be free to create and inspire. Be free to do whatever it is that gives you hope, inspiration, and passion. This will not only change the face of aging in America, but can also revolutionize the country as a whole. Forget the stereotypes—consider it an exercise in health!

CHAPTER 2.
MORE PASSION – THE ROAD TO HAPPINESS

Why passion? Honestly, passion is a word that only recently worked its way into my life. I usually associated passion with lust or desire and typically relegated it to the bedroom. But lately I've realized that passion is so much more than an amorous emotion. Passion in the bedroom is only the beginning. What about a *passion for life*? Or a *passion for health*? Or a *passion for work*? Passion is something that can bubble in any situation—if you let it.

My newfound focus on passion is the byproduct of decades of caring for older adults. While helping thousands of patients navigate the aging process—and embarking on it myself—I finally realized that the line separating those who age well from those who age poorly often has little to do with medicine. It's rarely just about fitness or nutrition or the absence of illness. Those who age well have more than health; they have passion.

Those who age well exude passion toward everything—the good and the bad, sickness and health. They defy stereotypes, break molds, and squeeze every ounce out of life. They *choose* to be passionate about every aspect of life. They choose to enjoy the little, mundane things in life, because they understand that every moment is precious and not to be wasted.

The first step in Dr. David's longevity plan is to find *more* passion. Passion is the road to happiness. Cultivate passion for everything you do, and you will certainly live a healthier, happier, and more independent life.

Finding your passion

Most of us never had the luxury to be passionate about what we do, where we live, or even how we live. The pressures and obligations of life can keep you in a rut, where each day is more about survival than enjoyment. Happiness exists mainly in the future—some holiday or event to look forward to. The in-between times, the mundane times, are what make us appreciate the happy times.

But with this sort of outlook, it's easy to get weighed down and never experience happiness in the day-to-day. You lose your passion for life! What's more, you'll wake up at 65 and realize that life has passed you by!

If you want to be healthy and happy at 95, you have to create your own happiness, now. *This* is where passion comes in. As Joseph Campbell said, "Follow your bliss. Wherever you are—if you are following your bliss, you are enjoying that refreshment, that life within you, all the time." Finding your passion is the road to happiness at any age.

Passion can come in many forms, and your source of passion will be different from mine. If you love to dance, dance. If you love to paint, paint. If you love to go on walks—do that, too. Whatever it is—from starting a business to learning healthy cooking, from lobbying congress to caring for your grandchildren—passion is a unique expression of who you are.

If you are following your passion, engaging passion in every aspect (both the good and the bad), you will be a healthier person. But beware: living a passionate life is not about doing whatever you like, freeing yourself from obligation, or escaping from the challenges of life. Instead, it's about identifying your own passions and giving yourself to them full-force. It's about eliminating the unnecessary stressors of life, taking an honest look at your future, and determining what it will take for you to age well.

Life will still have ups and downs, successes and failures. But by pursuing your passion and applying passion to every element of your life, health and happiness will follow.

Cultivating your passion

We all have passion within us. The challenge is to find it, cultivate it, and have the courage to follow it. Consider these three tips to cultivating your passion:

1. **Take an honest look at yourself.** We continue to grow and change at every stage in life. After a certain point—whether it's 55, 65, or 95—there comes a time when you must look

inward and make an honest assessment of where you are, where you are going, and where you want to be. With more years behind you than in front, these are important questions to ask. The answers may be predictable or surprising, but they will certainly reveal a unique truth about your own state of happiness and passion. By being honest, you'll unveil the path you most want to follow.

2. **Be grateful.** Wherever you find yourself in life, learn to be grateful for everything. Be grateful for your life, your health, yourfamily,andyourcommunity.Begratefulforthechallenges you face and the failures you've experienced, because you'll learn more from challenge and failure than from any success. Approach each moment in your day with gratitude, both the good and the bad. By doing so, you'll learn to see the positive in everything.

Be prepared to change. Change is an inevitable component of everyone's life. When you're trying to cultivate your passion, you must have the courage to change if necessary. It may mean changing your habits, your desires, your actions, or your attitude. Whatever it is, following your passion usually requires some change. Every day I marvel sometimes at the sheer stupidity of giving up true security and taking on a new career. However for me the choice was never in doubt and I am comfortable that the choice was right for me. After a year it all seems to be falling into place

Start from here.
This is the starting point of *your* Longevity Plan. Every element of this book should be considered with passion in mind; each step is another piece of the puzzle. Use them to find your own passion for life, love, health and happiness. It's the key to staying young at heart.

CHAPTER 3
MORE PEACE AND *LESS* STRESS!

In the last decade, the country has been on a path to democratize health, bringing it down from a scholarly level and allowing the average, interested American to access huge amounts of medical information. Today, every major news channel has a "medical correspondent," newspapers have entire sections dedicated to health, the internet has millions of websites to quench your thirst for information, and magazine racks are lined with publications that offer new health tips.

The end result is both fantastic and completely overwhelming. Sorting through the current health advice is a totally daunting task because the recommendations continue to change! What seemed right yesterday may seem wrong today. With the aging baby boomers acutely aware of their health, navigating the avalanche of health tips can be very stressful. Pile that on to the stress we already feel at work, at home, and in our relationships, and being healthy becomes more of chore than a passion

If there is one grain of wisdom I could pass on to everyone I meet, it is to *stop stressing*! We stress about our weight, our health, our families, our jobs, our nation, our faith, and anything else that varies, changes, or leaves uncertainty. As a nation, we have got to learn to relax: the stress is killing us.

The second step in Dr. David's Longevity Plan is *more* peace and *less* stress.

Living a truly healthy life begins with *calming down*. Find peace with where you are right now and learn to relax. Too much stress causes heart disease, anxiety, high blood pressure, and many other chronic conditions. Managing your stress and making room for peace in your life is just as important to your health as exercise or nutrition. But stress management is a skill. You must to *learn* to reduce stress; it's not a simple task. By freeing yourself from stress, you will be well on your way to a healthier, happier life.

Finding my own sense of peace.

For me, understanding the role of stress and health has been some-what of a challenge. For a large part of my life, I lived with a high degree of stress … and I liked it! Running a department of geriatrics and developing a world-renowned Institute on Aging offered con-stant challenges and pressures. It was only a matter of time before my stress caught up to me—and, 10 years ago, it did.

At 55 years old, I was on the brink of creating a freestanding center for geriatric care and research that could revolutionize the way we approached and understood aging. It was a very exciting—and stressful—time. We had just submitted a 33 million-dollar grant to the Donald W. Reynolds Foundation, which, if awarded, would be the largest single grant ever given to the medi-cal school. I was wrought with anxiety. A few months before the grants were to be announced, I agreed to participate in a whirl-wind lecture tour through Asia. Over two weeks, I visited Hong Kong, Taiwan, Thailand, and Malaysia, lecturing in a different town each night. Between lecturing, traveling, and being entertained by my hosts, I was exhausted. To sum it up, my "vacation" went some-thing like this: I ate, slept, spoke, and rushed my way through Asia. At the end of the two weeks, I gave my last lecture and finally be-gan the arduous, 40-hour trip home. A day later and on my way to the office with severe jet lag, nausea, and discomfort, I had a heart attack.

I'd like to say that the heart attack was a wake-up call for me, but it wasn't. My physicians had to remove the phone from my room to keep me from working in the hospital bed! Eight weeks later, I was back at work with a vengeance. I was so intently focused on the grant request that I nearly forgot about the heart attack altogether. Rumors were flying that the foundation had chosen to support another institution and I honestly believed that my chances were growing slimmer by the day. Finally I got a call from the chancellor of our institution. His message simply said, "I have heard from the foundation, be in my office at 9:00 am." It was then 7:00 am! My mouth was dry, my chest was tight, and my heart raced. Fearing the worst, I remember saying to my wife, "This is the worst month of my life." When I finally made it to his office, it was good news! The Institute on Aging would become a reality.

You might think that I felt a huge sense of relief and basked in the glory of our success … and I did, for a minute. But the feeling of victory was fleeting compared to the heightened pressure of actually completing the project. Within days, I started to run again, even more intent on reaching new heights and achieving new successes. I barely had a chance to stop and catch my breath.

The highs and lows of those few months took a sizeable toll on my health. Sleeping was difficult, exercise impossible, and food offered the only comfort. Add that all to my cardiologist's prescription to "take it easy" and "reduce stress," and I was truly a walking time bomb.

I had to change something, but I didn't really know what to do. One day as I was riding the elevator to my own doctor's appointment, I saw a flyer for a new health education course, "Learning to Cope with Cancer." I immediately thought, "If they can teach someone to cope with cancer, surely they can teach me to cope with stress." That decision changed my life forever.

Over the next several months, I saw a wonderful therapist regularly. He name is Stephanie Simonton and she is a world famous academician who has written the book on teaching patients to cope with cancer. We slowly unpacked every element of my stress from work to home. I never really understood how little peace I had! With each session, I learned new coping skills to help manage the many challenges in life. Slowly, I opened my eyes to the amazingly powerful effect of stress on one's health.

During our sessions, Stephanie taught me the mechanics of reducing stress, but most importantly she helped me respect the value of peace in my daily life. I learned to let go and resolved to be a better father, husband, son, and boss. In the end, I came out of the process a thoroughly changed human being. I was more effective at my job, kinder to my children, and happier with myself.

Today, over ten years later, I continue to seek peace in every element of my life. It's important that we learn to understand the incredible value of peace in work, in relationships, and with ourselves.

In order to incorporate more peace and less stress in your life, let's first look at exactly what stress is and how it affects our bodies.

What is stress?

<u>The science of stress</u>

Stress is a natural and vital element of the human condition. At its core, stress is the main cause of the fight-or-flight response. When faced with a stressful situation—whether physical, emotional, or psychological—humans and animals respond with a heightened sense of urgency, power, and capabilities. Think about it: prepare to run a 100-meter hurdle, take a standardized test, give a concert, or take on a serious confrontation, and your body responds! Hormones rush in to save the day and you feel an increased sense of awareness, your brain is sharper, and your entire body tenses in preparation. At this sort of heightened state, humans can conquer seemingly impossible challenges, like lifting a car off a trapped child or rushing into a burning building to save a loved one. Your body's natural reaction to stress takes over and can literally protect you from disaster. This is what is supposed to happen. But—fortunately or unfortunately—we no longer live in a time of fight-or-flight. Stress today is not usually one major event to which we must respond. Rather, stress is an ongoing, subversive, and very dangerous problem in the average American's life. Many of us live in a perpetual state of heightened awareness from which we never "come down."

But what actually happens in the body during times of stress?

In times of acute stress, your body launches an intricate series of reactions and changes to help you cope with conflict. Messages from your brain go to your vascular system through the autonomic nervous system, which controls all involuntary functions such as breathing, heart rate, bowel and bladder movement, etc. When exposed to a serious threat, a message is carried through the brain to a tiny area called the anterior hypothalamus, activating the autonomic nervous system, which in turn sends signals throughout the body. Adrenalin and noradrenalin are released from the nerve endings; they cause your heart to beat faster, dilate blood vessels, and regulate body temperature through increased sweating. Extra blood is then diverted to your muscles in order to allow for maximum function and strength. Simultaneously, glucose is released from energy stores to provide that extra boost during stressful times. All of these functions prepare you for the fight-or-flight reaction.

This orchestra of physiologic responses from the autonomic nervous system occurs within a matter of seconds. Any time a stressful situation lasts a few minutes or less, such as running a 100-meter race or quickly swerving away from an oncoming car, the body relies completely on the autonomic nervous system. However, in cases where the stress lasts for a longer amount of time, the brain simultaneously signals the adrenal gland to release a flood of hormones that allow the body to maintain a heightened level of function. If the stressor continues for hours, like running a marathon or being in a very stressful situation for a prolonged time, then the hormones from the adrenal gland take over.

The main hormone released by the adrenal gland is *cortisol*, which plays a key role in metabolism to provide the body with as much fuel possible. It mobilizes all the body's stores of glucose, and simultaneously breaks down fat and protein to form even more glucose. (Remember, glucose is sugar, the easiest, most available, and rapid source of energy.) It also opposes the function of insulin, keeping the body's blood sugar high. Cortisol suppresses the immune system, helps to prevent allergies, and suppresses inflammation. Ultimately, cortisol helps focus all of the body's activity on dealing with the stressful insult.

In addition to cortisol, the adrenal gland releases *vasopressin*, a hormone that promotes fluid retention, constricts blood vessels and causes the blood pressure to rise. Finally *thyroxin* is released from the thyroid gland to cause an increase in metabolism, which contributes to the feeling of being frightened, raising the heart rate, and causing the bowels and bladder to hyper function.

This well-orchestrated and highly strategic process calls on the very innate function of protecting us from injury, whether real or perceived. Ultimately, dealing with stress in this basic manner can be very positive and healthy. It even can be beneficial, allowing you to perform to best of your ability. Consider athletes like Peyton Manning or Tiger Woods who rely on their body's ability to function well during stressful situations. It helps raise them above their competition.

Stress and disease

In times of stress, this chain reaction of internal events is all part of your body's natural response and it's meant to be used! You are supposed to jump away from that car, flee from a predator, or scream at an opponent. Those sort of physical reactions allow you to release that pent-up energy and bring your body back down to a regulated state. Remember, anything that goes up must come down. Your body and its reaction to external stress is no exception.

When maintained too long and without any physical or emotional release, each of the positive stress responses has an equally negative effect. If stress persists, the body becomes fatigued and the initial benefits become negative (figure 1). With chronic stress—which can occur over days, months and years—over-functioning of the autonomic nervous system causes a variety of health problems, including heart disease, diabetes, cancer, and other serious conditions.

Let's break it down piece by piece to see exactly how the stress response can negatively affect your body. First, increased vasopressin leads to fluid retention and high blood pressure. Increased cortisol production leads to a higher risk of diabetes, increased risk of cholesterol deposits in the blood vessels, and can contribute to weight gain or weight loss. Just as importantly, it contributes to long-term suppression of the immune system that can cause cancer, increased risk of infections, and a number of autoimmune diseases such as rheumatoid arthritis and lupus.

A diagram indicating the relationship between stress and disease is illustrated in figure 2. As you can see, if the stress becomes chronic, your body enters a phase of nervous and endocrine over-stimulation that has negative effects on your health, your sense of well-being, your relationships, and your ability to succeed in nearly every aspect of life. Any number of physical and emotional conditions can be aggravated or caused by stress, including anxiety, depression, irritable bowel syndrome, insomnia, fibromyalgia, substance abuse, obesity, and many others.

The mainstream community of physicians has taken quite a long time to understand the impact of stress on health. Much of what we know about stress comes from the work of Dr. Hans Selye, one of the true giants in medical science. Selye was the first person to use the word "stress."

Through research with animals, Selye showed that stressful environments contributed to clear pathological changes in health and behavior. When the animals were exposed to an acute stressful situation, such as blaring light, loud noise, or severe heat or cold, they developed an array of conditions including stomach ulcers, enlargement of the adrenal glands, and declines in lymph nodes, the core of the immune system. But when exposed to continued stressful situations over a prolonged period of time, the animals developed chronic illnesses, including heart disease, strokes, renal failure, and immune disorders such as rheumatoid arthritis and increased susceptibility to infections.

In addition to contributing to a host of chronic diseases, there is even evidence at the cell level that long-term stress has a detrimental impact on your health. In fact, chronic stress may actually accelerate the aging process!

Recently, researchers have been increasingly interested in the idea of one's "biologic age." Your biologic age is determined by the health of your cells. Cells that have been exposed to a high degree of stress or damage do not function as well and may contribute to many age-related diseases. A person who has been unhealthy for the majority of his or her life will likely have more cell damage—and therefore age "more quickly"—than someone who has led a relatively clean life.

One of the most accurate measures of biologic aging is found at the end of each chromosome in an area called the *telomere*.

With each cell division, the telomere shortens. Once the telomere shortens to a critical level, the cell loses its ability to divide … and quickly dies. In animal models, telomere shortening is a sensitive marker of the animal's biologic age.

In an elegant research study published by the National Academy of Sciences, scientists from the University of Utah, Vanderbilt, Ohio State University, and the University of California at San Francisco assessed the impact of chronic stress on mothers caring for ill children. The stressed mothers' telomeres in immune cells were much shorter than normal, which was accompanied by decline in the cell's ability to function. In addition, there was evidence of increased antioxidant stress that caused even more cell damage. The chronic stress appears to accelerate the aging process, which in turn causes age-related declines to occur at an earlier age.

The bottom line: Chronic stress makes you sick, old, and unhappy!

Why are we so stressed?

Who isn't stressed? Everyone I know feels stress, whether they're 25, 55, or 85. With each new decade, it seems that the stressors change and evolve. What stressed you out at 30 probably doesn't stress you out at 60. What stresses you out today probably won't stress you out ten years from now!

Ultimately, we live in a very stressful society. The American Dream and its promise of independence created a culture where *we* were completely responsible for our own success. As a result, we define ourselves by what we achieve. By and large, Americans believe that the harder you work, the better and more successful you will be. We work harder and longer than any other nation in the world. What's more, we continue to raise the bar on what it means to be successful. No matter where someone is on the socio-economic scale, we tend to think that they can always do more, achieve more, and see more measures of success. We push and push … and then push some more.

Many Americans today don't feel productive unless they're stressed! Stress at work and at home has become the norm. We don't know what to do without pressure to perform. What's more, we've become so conditioned to feel stressed at work or at home that some of us feel totally uncomfortable *without* it.

America's Stressors

Today, stress comes in many forms—whether at work, at home, or simply from images on the television. We are exposed to stressful situations over and over again and it continues to have a negative impact on our health.

When you think about stress in the context of the American experience, it likely comes as no surprise that for 75% of Americans—myself included—work and money are the two major sources of stress. For me, at 66, retirement is nowhere in sight, so the issue of job stress continues to impact my life and the lives of my family members.

According to the National Institute for Occupational Safety and Health (NIOSH), over 40% of employees say that their work is extremely stressful. One in four Americans maintains that his or her job is the most stressful part of life. Over 75% of people say their stress level is rising and 26% of us are burned out. *Burned out!* "Burnout" is the opposite of healthy.

Job stress causes unhealthy ramifications across the spectrum, from productivity and absenteeism to violence and depression. Many American employees work long hours at a fast pace. Expectations are high, deadlines are tight, and there is little or no leeway for mistakes. As a result, many workers experience physiologic effects of a stressful job, including back pain, headache, anxiety, and severe fatigue. This contributes in turn to reduced productivity, increased mistakes, and more accidents. An estimated 80% of all accidents are stress-related.

In addition to the emotional and physical effects for employees, job stress takes a huge financial toll on American employers. From lost productivity to increases in health care costs and insurance, it is estimated that work-related stress costs American industries 300 billion dollars annually.

A worker with high stress is two times more likely to miss five or more days of work. In 1993, researchers found that one million workers stay home each day due to stress, which translates into 550 million lost days due to absenteeism. And recent statistics show that employee absenteeism is rising dramatically! A recent survey of 800,000 workers from over 300 major companies revealed that the number of workers who called in sick tripled from 1996 and 2000. If one million employees stayed home in 1993, how many do you think stay home today?

Not surprisingly, perhaps the most devastating financial effect of workplace stress comes from increased healthcare costs. Research shows that 60 to 90% of doctor visits are stress-related. Considering the cost of health insurance is the fastest growing component of business expenses, the effect of poorly managed job stress is enormous.

While stress may originate at work, its impact on the home life is very serious. Today most couples are part of the workforce, and each partner brings his or her unique stressors to the relationship. Worries about finances, job insecurity, and performance all take a tremendous toll and marriages and children. With 50% of marriages ending in divorce, it's not a stretch to assume that poorly managed stress is a major culprit.

When you're not coping well with stress, it's virtually impossible to see beyond your own personal problems. When it comes to relationships, individual stress is often released on your partner, even if the true cause of your stress is miles away. Every conflict is personalized, forcing you to always assume a defensive stance. In these dually stressed relationships, miscommunication is rampant. We fight too much, take each other for granted, take out our frustrations on those we love the most, and test relationships to the limit.

But what about stress from other areas of life besides work? If 50% of Americans place work as the number-one stressor in life, then 50% of us have other, non-work sources of stress. Family relationships are likely high on the list, especially as both our children *and* our parents age.

For baby boomers in the "sandwich generation," I predict that the stress of an aging parent will soon rise to the top of the stress list. It's estimated that 21% of the American population provides care for an older adult. In the next 30 years, that number will skyrocket.

As a geriatrician, I have seen thousands of children deal with the challenges of caregiving. But only recently, as my own mother became increasing frail, have I truly understood the turmoil of a becoming your parent's parent.

My mother's annual visit to the United States recently ended. Unfortunately, this trip was more eventful—and stressful—than most. As soon as she arrived in the country, my mother was sick. She developed a markedly elevated blood pressure that was difficult to get under control. She felt ill most of the time and simply was not up to the task of going out, seeing friends, or doing much of anything. Overall, she seemed quite a bit frailer than usual and, after a long three weeks, she vowed this would be her last trip overseas.

As a son, these changes in my mother were difficult to see. But as a geriatrician I knew what was on the horizon. With each passing year, my mother has an increasingly high chance of becoming dependent. Living 10,000 miles away does not make this an easy discussion. I am helpless, as is my youngest brother and my eldest sister. Only my sister Jocelyn remains in South Africa. Luckily, she and my mom are very close, making her the natural caregiver. Although she has offered to have my mom move in with her and her husband, my mother refuses to even consider it.

My mother wants no part of our plans for her eventual dependence. She never wants to be a burden on her children. "Thank God I can take care of myself," she tells me. "If ever I can't, just shoot me!" Ridiculous as it is, many of my patients feel the same way. Our parents want lifelong freedom and independence ... just as we do. Unfortunately, this creates a very stressful dynamic between parent and child. Although everyone wants the best, the plan for how to get there often differs greatly.

Children want their parents to be safe—to move out of the house, to stop driving, to hire a nurse. Parents want to be independent; they hate the idea of leaving their home, abhor the prospect of not driving, and simply refuse to share the burden of an aging body with anyone. Over and over again the same argument erupts and leaves neither parent nor child happy. But the stress of caregiving extends well beyond the parent-child relationship. Caregivers must balance their work, their own children, their spouses, and their own happiness. Caregivers are pulled in every direction and have little time to recover. The stress is virtually endless. Caregivers of a dependent loved have an eight-fold higher risk of developing illness.

We don't know how to cope…
Regardless of what the greatest stressor may be, the majority of Americans simply do not know how to cope with stress. This is probably why stress doesn't end with retirement. Stress is not just about a job or a situation; it exists everywhere, and until you learn to use positive coping mechanisms, you will never be stress-free.

More and more evidence shows that, as a nation, we are not dealing with stress well. According to a recent survey of the American Psychological Association, 78% of Americans admit to using poor coping skills when it comes to stress. Too much stress may cause you to overeat or under-eat. It may make you more prone to lash out at others and cause unnecessary conflicts. Stress may push you to seek mindless activities like watching television or playing video games. At its worst, too much stress can lead to abuse of alcohol or drugs.

Let's go back to the workplace for a minute. A Gallup survey conducted in 2000 indicated that more and more employees turn to violence and hostility to manage stress at work. The data is truly astounding: 14% of employees felt like striking a coworker, 25% felt like screaming or shouting at work, 9% were aware of a violent act at work, and 28% had been threatened some time in the last year. 20 people are killed at work each week, 18,000 non-violent crimes are committed in the workplace, and over one million assaults occur annually. Desk rage, phone rage and road rage are now part of everyday language!

Clearly, this is a major indication that we are reaching our limit on how much stress any one person can handle.

Our inability to manage stress at work is rippling out to every element of our lives. We have difficulty balancing work and home. Problems at work inevitably cause problems at home, and vice versa. Work suffers, relationships suffer, health suffers, and the end result is a never-ending cycle where stress begets stress and peace is nonexistent.

Learning to cope

The world will never be a stress-free place. We will always face challenging and stressful situations. But it is not the stress that causes problems. It is your reaction to stress that determines your health. Ultimately, this is the greatest challenge to our overall health and well-being.

There are many different coping skills to help you manage your stress. Whether it's finding a strong support network, embracing your faith, or simply taking more time for yourself, stress management is somewhat of a personal process. However, there are two main techniques that helped me reduce stress and seek peace: mindfulness-based stress reduction (MBSR) and guided imagery.

Guided imagery

When I had my heart attack, the first way my therapist helped reduce stress was through a 15-minute guided imagery tape, to which I was instructed to listen every day. This was my first introduction to meditation and, despite a healthy amount of skepticism, I was so desperate for relief that I embraced it wholeheartedly.

Guided imagery relies on your mind's ability to affect your body. There is an incredible interplay between mental health and physical health, so guided imagery offers an avenue to help you tap in your subconscious thoughts and emotions. Imagery is used to create a state of relaxation that bears a close similarity to self-hypnosis. Somewhat easier than sitting cross-legged in a silent room, guided imagery tapes give you a script to follow with your mind.

Guided imagery can be used for a variety of reasons, from relaxation to healing to motivation. Depending on the goal, the imagery will vary. However, guided imagery almost always begins by helping you focus on your breath and conscious relaxation of every muscle group. It involves moving ever more downward as you become increasingly relaxed. For example, you imagine yourself moving down a hill and with each step downward you become more and more relaxed, more and more at peace.

Once you've reached a level of deep relaxation, you will hear a series of directions that help you imagine a place that brings you peace, comfort, and a sense of calm. You may be asked to visualize smells in that place and become so familiar with it that you may easily withdraw there. The guided imagery may lead you to imagine yourself surrounded by a golden light with healing powers. If the goal is relaxation, being surrounded by this light will bring calm. If it is pain relief, the powerful image will focus on the area of pain. Some imagery even suggests that a powerful force provides support for and assists in helping curing disease, such as fighting a cancer or easing inflammation.

Whatever your needs, you can find a guided imagery script to help. A script developed by Harold H. Benjamin, Ph.D can be found in Section D of the appendix. This script is generic and includes examples of how it may be used to help with pain management, stress management, and coping with illness.

Mindfulness
Guided imagery was my first introduction to meditation and relaxation, but mindfulness helped lay the foundation for lifelong peace.

Mindfulness is an extremely powerful and effective technique to manage stress. Rooted in Buddhism (though not limited to Buddhists!), mindfulness is the process of being fully awake and present to each moment in life. Through mindfulness, you can learn to appreciate every element of your day-to-day events, from the momentous to the mundane. By increasing your awareness and being more mindful of your own thoughts, feelings, and reactions, you can better understand how you deal with stress. In doing so, you can develop a more solid perspective on life's many challenges.

Mindfulness made its debut on the medical scene through the work of Dr. Jon Kabat-Zinn from the University of Massachusetts. Kabat-Zinn developed an eight-week course entitled Mindfulness-Based Stress Reduction that leveraged mindfulness to help individuals manage pain, stress, or anxiety. Over the years, this course has grown and expanded throughout the country, helping Americans of all ages learn to develop healthier ways to reduce stress and improve health.

In order to educate about mindfulness and health, Dr. Kabat-Zinn has published numerous research papers demonstrating the powerful benefit of mindfulness training on controlling chronic pain, from back pain to joint pain, irritable bowel syndrome to fibromyalgia. He has also shown that mindfulness training improves self-esteem and reduces anxiety. Research published in 2007 in the journal *Arthritis Care* showed a powerful beneficial effect of mindfulness meditation in reducing the symptoms of rheumatoid arthritis. It has also been linked to reducing the risk of heart disease and high blood pressure. The National Institutes of Health recently undertook a large clinical trial examining the role of mindfulness meditation in reducing the risk of a heart attack in patients with proven heart disease. This study commenced in 2003 and results should be available shortly.

Though I had heard of Dr. Kabat-Zinn, I was first introduced to mindfulness and MBSR through a colleague at the Institute on Aging, Dr. Sandy Pope. Throughout her time at the Institute on Aging, Sandy offered MBSR courses for our patients and the community at large. Sandy and her assistant, Mary, always seemed so content with themselves and I never really understood what the whole "mindfulness" thing was about.

So, one day, I went to Sandy and asked her to explain it to me. I was ready to embark on a new phase of my own pursuit of peace. She told me that most of us live our days with an endless array of thoughts, feelings, or ideas streaming through our brain. These thoughts can be good or bad, calming or stressful. Whatever they are, they generally keep us from engaging in the present moment. One thought leads to another and then to another—and before you know it the thoughts have led you off in a totally different direction and you've missed whatever happened in front of you! At best, this causes us to "drift off" for a moment. At worst, it allows us to totally misunderstand or misinterpret a situation or scenario. By learning to be more mindful, she said, we can learn to respond better and more appropriately to any challenge, especially stressful ones.

Suddenly, at that very moment, I got it! She was talking about *me*. I constantly have new thoughts and ideas running through my brain. My children even think I have attention-deficit disorder! I realized that I spent a majority of my time in my head—and there's very little peace in that. At that moment, I recognized my own constant flow of distracting ideas and feelings. That recognition *was* mindfulness. It was like an "ah-ha" moment in my path to more peace. That day, I signed up for her course.

The eight-week Mindfulness-Based Stress-Reduction class was an intensive study of meditation and awareness. All participants in an MBSR course begin with learning the power of the breath. Your breath is a constant guide that helps bring you back to the present moment. By taking a minute to notice your breath—the in and out flow—you momentarily stop the cycle of distracting thoughts. When you find yourself slipping back into any thoughts or feelings, you simply notice your breath again without judgment. You'll find yourself in an ongoing process of coming in and out of presence. But in those moments of mindfulness, you can exist in a completely present state where neither the past nor the future exists. It's a little slice of peace.

Focusing on the breath and learning to sit quietly in meditation is the first step in a gradual journey to true mindfulness, peace, tranquility and understanding. With each week of the MBSR course, I learned new skills and tools that add to an overall sense of peace and well-being. It's truly amazing how simply being present can impact your health!

Learning the skills of meditation is a vital element of reducing stress. There are many different forms of meditation and MBSR is not the only avenue to develop these skills. However, the process of committing to practice is an essential component of long-term success. Remember, seeking peace and reducing stress is a process and a journey—it takes patience and practice.

12 steps to *more* peace

Stress management—like exercise, eating right, or navigating the health system—is a serious and challenging component of health promotion. It's a skill that can be learned, but it does take work. After years of therapy, and then passing that information along to my patients, I've found that there are key steps that can help anyone achieve greater peace.

1. Passion! (again)

With stress management, it all comes back to passion. Tackle life with passion. Throw love and energy into everything you do. From work to play, it is critical that you love every minute of the day and treat it with respect. The more you embrace and enjoy your life at home, work, and play, the more at peace you will be. At any age or any stage in life, open yourself up to follow what you love most.

2. Put yourself first.

Be honest with yourself—and others—about what you need. Give yourself the leeway to be first once in a while. This applies to all aspects of your life, including the time you spend with your family. If you have concerns, learn to be honest, discuss your feelings openly, and actively look for opportunities to improve your situation. You can never find peace if you constantly feel unsatisfied in a job or a relationship. By putting yourself first, you will actually be better for everyone around you. This is not a selfish task, but rather a necessary component of being truly peaceful.

3. Be kind to your body and seek health.

Your health is precious, and nothing is more important than taking care of yourself. A healthy body is going to be much more prepared to handle stress. Follow the steps of this book, and you'll find that each step is another component in seeking peace! Have love in your life, embrace your faith, and treat yourself kindly. Eat right, exercise, and be an empowered consumer of health care. Always maintain good health habits.

Following the basic elements of a healthy life can help you identify positive coping skills instead of negative ones. Exercise is a great stress-reliever. Listen to your body and don't burn the candle at both ends. When you're tired, you probably need to sleep.

4. Don't take yourself too seriously and learn to laugh.
Anyone who has the capacity to laugh at himself or herself and see humor in any situation is bound to be a more peaceful and relaxed person. Voltaire said eloquently, "The art of medicine consists of keeping the patient amused while nature heals the disease." In other words, don't stress about it! Your body has an incredible ability to heal itself, and the more lighthearted you are, the better.

5. Be kind—to yourself and to others.
Developing healthy interpersonal relationships is a huge component of living a stress-free life. But remember: it begins with you. Be kind to yourself and you can learn to be kind to others as well. Be vulnerable, open, and honest. Once you open yourself up to other people, you simply cannot be a hard-ass anymore. (And being a hard-ass isn't healthy!)

6. Learn to say no.
Many of us simply take on too much … myself included! I took quite a long time learning to refuse opportunity, delegate tasks, and simply make time for myself. Remember, the greater the responsibility, the more important it is to not take everything on yourself. Numerous studies have shown that the most successful people are not that busy.

7. Don't let the little things get to you.
It's amazing how often we get upset over the smallest things. Remember what is important and put your challenges into

perspective. Usually, getting upset about little things is a byprod-uct of a bigger problem. Seek the source of your issue.

8. Learn how to handle conflict.
Perhaps the best lesson I learned from my therapist was how to handle conflict. We have a tendency to either confront disagree-ments aggressively or bury them in our mind and stew. Neither is of great value. When you find yourself in a challenging situation, take a moment to breathe and try to find the core reason for your conflict. It's often not what's on the surface.

When dealing with interpersonal conflict, discuss your concerns in a calm environment and, whatever you do, avoiding a shouting match. Try and induce sympathy in the person you are confronting and avoid accusations. Never attack and always relate to the way the prob-lem has negatively affected you. Choose to collaborate rather than agitate.

9. Learn to forgive.
Forgiveness plays a major role in promoting health and assuring a long and independent life. It rids you of resentment, hostility, and negative thoughts that can eat away at you. Whether it is by em-bracing your faith, calling on your inner strength, or seeking help from others, having the capacity to forgive and let go, allows heal-ing, growth, comfort, and peace.

10. Maintain your boundaries between work and home.
Nothing is worse than coming home after a stressful day and let-ting your work issues affect your home life. Try to come up with a ritual that helps you separate the challenges between work and home. It may mean taking a few moments of silence in your car before you head home. Or it could be taking a walk each day after work. Whatever it is, find something that allows your mind to focus on what's right in front of you, *not* what you left at work or at home, or what you'll confront tomorrow.

11. Recognize what stresses you out.

We all have certain triggers that can send us off. Find out what your trigger is and try to address it. Each time you feel that thing happen—whatever it is—stop and breathe. Try to relax and approach the situation anew.

There are aspects of our lives that will always be stressful. Whether it's caring for an aging parent or coping with illness, managing money or simply talking to your sister, stress will always exist. By being honest and recognizing whatever stresses you out, you will be able to cope more effectively.

12. Stop. Breathe. Seek peace.

Learning to unwind and seek true and inner peace will save your life. Whenever you find yourself stressed or revved up, stop and breathe. Notice your breath. Find peace in this present moment. Doing so will bring you back, calm you down, and provide a little extra room to be honest.

Stop stressing

The message is simple: *Stress is bad.* Chronic stress is unhealthy, unproductive, and eats away at your personal well-being. Living a healthy life must begin by reducing your stress. Only then can you really free yourself to take on the many other challenges of pursing health.

Just like diet, exercise and a visit to your doctor, stress management is not passive: it involves active and often difficult approaches to achieve your goal. It takes work and is a skill that can be learned. These twelve tips are only guidelines to get you started on a path to a more stress-free life.

CHAPTER 4
LOVE MORE

I'd hazard to guess that most doctors (including me, in my first years of practice!) don't give a lot of mental energy to their patients' private lives. They aren't about to use up valuable time asking about relationships, whether or not patients are dating or have a partner, or if they're happy at home. Modern medicine is all about tests, exams, and physical findings. Things like love and contentment can't be detected in a blood test or plotted on a graph. So doctors don't bother with them.

But how can a doctor possibly understand your health if he or she doesn't know what goes on outside the clinic doors? Your health—not just your condition or illness—is about *every* element of your life. As a geriatrician, it's absolutely imperative that I know my patients as people, not just bodies with medical problems or diseases. As we age, those "non-important" factors that most physicians ignore (like love, community, and relationships) can have a greater impact on your health than family history or genetics.

It makes sense. Who cares about heart disease when you're lonely? How can you strive to exercise or eat right when your marriage is bad? With each passing decade, one thing becomes increasingly clear: you cannot be healthy without love in your life. What's more, love is potent predictor of longevity. People who love more live longer.

The third step in Dr. David's Longevity Plan is to love *more*. Those of us who learn to love—and to love passionately—will live a healthier, happier, and longer life. Love in any form (whether it's from a child, spouse, friend, or pet) can truly transform your life and your health.

Love is clearly a multi-faceted issue. So in order to help you understand love and its affect on health, we're going to approach it from two angles. First, we'll discuss love, intimate relationships, and how to maintain a healthy, loving relationship. Second, we'll look at the power of having a community of love and the impact of social connectedness on your health.

Let's begin by understanding how love became a core component of my prescription for lifelong health.

A physician's perspective

I began my training as a geriatrician over 25 years ago. Newly relocated to Little Rock, Arkansas, I was a young physician and researcher in the very new field of geriatrics. Over the years, I became well versed on the unique needs of older adults. From evaluation and diagnosis to medications and treatment, caring for an aging body was certainly an acquired skill. But it took me quite a while to incorporate a more comprehensive approach to health, one that included the "softer side" of medicine. When I look back on how I've grown as a physician and a teacher, the greatest lessons have been beyond the mechanics of geriatric medicine.

When it came to understanding the power of love and health, the lesson was not learned from a textbook or research study (although there are countless scientific studies on the relationship between love and health). Rather, my patients taught me the *power* of love. I've never forgotten the couple that came into my office decades ago. These two people—completely comfortable with each other and so passionately in love—shaped the way I practice medicine.

At the time, I was still a young physician in my mid-40s and had a lot to learn from this elderly couple who had endured 50 years of marriage. Throughout their visit, it was obvious that they adored each other. Gently holding hands or exchanging a quick kiss, it was as though they'd just met … and yet they'd been together for decades! You don't see that kind of thing very often; not in the young, and certainly not in the very old. Yet here they were, these lovebirds, discussing some health problem or another, and clearly overjoyed to be spending yet another day in each other's presence.

When I think back to that visit, I still remember how healthy they seemed. Though they had their share of medical problems, as most 80-year-olds do, they were vibrant, energized, and happy to wake each day. Those two amazingly beautiful and loving adults pushed me, both as a person and as a physician, to look beyond the boundaries of medicine for my own prescription of healthy living.

Since that first couple, I have continued to meet thousands of men and women who thrive throughout their 70s, 80s, and 90s with love. Love does make them healthy, but it certainly tips the odds in their favor. These days, I routinely include questions about relationships when taking a health history. I can't change the way people live, but knowing if a patient is in a relationship provides some valuable hints about the overall state of health.

For married patients, the health benefits of love are pronounced. Married men and women have lower risks of heart disease and cancer. What's more, when they do get sick, they have a better prognosis. This is likely because married people see their doctors more regularly than single people. (The wife pushes the husband through the clinic doors!)

Beyond regular doctor visits, evidence suggests that marriage promotes other healthy activities as well. A large survey conducted in 1998 reported that older, married adults were more likely to exercise, wear seat belts, not smoke or drink, eat breakfast, and have their blood pressure checked than their unmarried peers.

Married men and women experience less depression than singles. They're less likely to abuse drugs or alcohol and their risk of suicide is much lower than that of their single counterparts. All in all, married people are happier by a significant margin than those who never married or are divorced or widowed.

A word about "relationships"
When speaking about long-term health, the term "relationships" is hardly limited to romantic involvements. It's true that men and women in long-term, committed relationships do better than those who are single. But so do unmarried couples. Close friendships— between men and women, women and women, and men and men—are also protective. And for many people, close companionship with a pet is just as good for long-term health as marriage!

Researchers who study the connections between relationships and health generally look at married couples. The very stability of their relationship makes them easy to track over long periods of time. But the evidence suggests that any stable relationship provides all, or nearly all, of the same benefits.

Any relationship is better than none. People who maintain active social networks, log many hours with friends and families, and keep their hearts open to others are far less likely to develop chronic or life-threatening diseases than those who shut themselves off from human contact. In our later years, the benefits are even more pronounced.

Remember, love doesn't discriminate. If you're lucky enough to have found your true soul-mate, the health odds are in your favor. If you have a best friend, someone you see often and with whom you're able to share emotional connections, the odds are *still* in your favor. Love can be expressed and received in so many different ways: between close friends, between parents and children, between teachers and students, and (of course) between doctors and patients. True intimacy, in whatever form, means sharing understanding, trust, and empathy. It means entering into the life of another and opening your life in turn.

Love, science, and longevity

When you have love in your life, your brain actually releases hormones that promote health. Over the years, researchers have become more aware of the unique science of love and the medical community has unearthed some very interesting findings on how love impacts health. Perhaps the most astounding effect of love on health relates to longevity: people who love more live longer!

Studies of men in long-term, loving, and monogamous relationships live an average of 10 years longer than men who divorced or were never married. Ten years! If a pharmaceutical company develops a drug that extends life by a year, they probably have a blockbuster product. Emotional commitment extends it by a *decade*. For women, the benefits aren't quite as dramatic, but still impressive. Married women live an average of three years longer than women who never married.

Here's another incredible statistic: In couples ages 70 years and older, if the wife dies first, the husband has a 30 percent chance of dying within a year of her death. If the husband dies first, the woman lives … well, just about forever. I know this kind of factoid sounds a little morbid, but it's impressive testimony to the profound effects of long-term relationships. It's also testimony to the fact that men, all clichés aside, have a far greater need for emotional connections than people normally assume.

Research has shown that people with strong social connections also benefit in the longevity arena. (I think it's fair to assume that someone with strong social connections has a lot of love in his or her life.) In one famous study, researchers tracked 4,725 residents of Alameda County, California. They found that those with the fewest social connections, including family members or close friends, had mortality rates that were two to three times higher than those with the most connections. Here's another way to look at this. People with a lot of close friends and social activities live an average of *nine years longer* than those without these connections.

Bad marriages work, too

Many of the protective effects of being in a committed relationship occur independently of happiness. This, to me, seems counterintuitive. Anyone who's been in an unhappy relationship (or around other people who are) knows how stressful the simplest interactions can be. You would think that people in unhappy relationships would get sicker than those who are single, divorced, or widowed.

Not true. More than half of couples surveyed report that they're dissatisfied with their marriage. As you'd expect, they have significantly more mental (and physical) problems than those who are happily married. And yet those dissatisfied couples that manage to stick it out show nearly all of the same benefits as those who were happy all along. This is probably because relationships invariably get better the longer people are together. (The truly bad relationships aren't likely to last.). In one survey, nearly 80 percent of those who rated their marriages as unhappy changed the ratings to "very happy" or "quite happy" when they were resurveyed five years later.

Beyond the science – my own path to health and love.
I've been talking about some of the quantifiable benefits of relationships, but the most powerful effects of love aren't so easily
measured. Well all know that love and companionship make our
lives stronger and more meaningful. That's not something you can
prove on a laboratory table.

I'd like to tell my own story. Not because my marriage is the
best in the world, but because it's like so many others: hardly ideal,
but far better than I could have hoped for. How time flies! It's hard
to imagine that my oldest child (from a previous marriage) is now
past 40, and that Francie and I recently celebrated our 32nd wed-
ding anniversary.

In many ways we're polar opposites. I am the man from Venus:
needy, affectionate, and loving intimacy. I love hugging, kissing,
and being close. Francie is a woman from Mars. She's headstrong
and sees things in black and white. She's a woman of strong prin-
ciples who has little sympathy for human frailties and weaknesses.
For Francie, public displays of affection are taboo and she is totally
uncomfortable when her personal space is invaded. On the surface she is very tough.

These emotional differences have led to quite a few rocky moments in the years we've been married. I am too demanding, she
says. She refuses to give, I say. In the early years—long gone, I'm
happy to say—my main approach to our differences was to fight
back with accusations, petulant outbursts, and personal attacks.
We had so many arguments that it was impossible to keep track
of what we were even fighting about. I was frustrated with her and
she was frustrated with me. I was immature and didn't understand
my wife very well (or, for that matter, women in general). This led to
extremes of male stupidity and irrational behavior, behavior that
I'll forever regret.

Despite some rough years—and they were *rough*—I always
knew that this unique woman was the true love of my life. The
core of our problems, which I didn't recognize until years later,
was my wish to change her to be more like me. The reality is that
that never works.

Fortunately, the therapy I received while learning to cope with stress spilled over into my relationship. While learning to be a more peaceful, vulnerable and loving person, I also began to understand my wife—an area of knowledge in which I was totally clueless.

Along the way, I realized the powerful role of love in promoting health and longevity. As my marriage improved, my well-being improved as well. Today? Our marriage is better than it's ever been. When I look at my wife, she takes my breath away. She's the only woman for me. And yet she's never changed. She's the same woman she always was. I'm the one who changed, who needed to change. I learned to compromise, to accept differences rather than fight through them, and to slow down professionally as well as personally. Finally, I am truly happy with what I have. But, man! It was a long time coming.

10 steps to making love last

The bonus of working with older patients is that I get a front-row seat for some truly amazing stories from folks who have been on Earth a lot longer than I have. Wisdom *does* accrue with age. Most of my patients are in their 70s, 80s, and 90s. More than a few of them have been with the same partners for almost as long as I've been alive. When you consider the astronomical rate of divorce in this country, that's the kind of inspiration we could all use more of.

Actually, inspiration is only part of the pleasure. Over the years, I've talked to literally thousands of couples. About their health issues, of course, but also about their marriages and relationships. They talk about things that worked and things that didn't. Mistakes they made, and how they got past them. How they communicate (or don't). No two stories are alike, and yet the underlying themes are surprisingly similar.

1. Stay faithful

This is no less true for monogamous singles than married couples. Infidelities—even those that don't necessarily involve sex—are the single biggest cause of crashed relationships.

If you're thinking about an infidelity, think again. Even if your marriage or relationship is less than ideal, you're a lot more likely to find long-term happiness if you work with your partner, take the conflicts head-on, and try mightily to work them out. It won't always work. Some marriages should end. But if that's the case, end it honestly. Don't do it by the back-door route of having an affair and waiting to get caught.

2. Talk and keep talking

Quite a few of the long-term couples I've known credit *total* communication for keeping them together. They have no secrets—and I mean none. They share everything: concerns about work, issues with children, personal details about friends, and so on. They're willing to criticize each other, safe in the knowledge that the criticism is meant to be constructive and helpful. The pages of their lives are always open.

Couples who don't communicate often and well invariably fall prey to misunderstandings, and misunderstandings lead to conflict and a failure of insight. I can't think of a better recipe for a poor relationship. Misunderstandings undermine more marriages than true conflicts. So lay your cards on the table, deal with small problems before they turn into disasters, and keep the channels of communication open.

3. Learn how to argue and negotiate

One of my patients told me about a really brutal fight she had with her husband. She was right to be angry, she told me, but she was mortified by how badly she handled it.

She'd spent a good part of the day, and much of the preceding week, getting ready for Christmas. Wrapping presents, baking, getting the house clean, the works. Her husband, to put it bluntly, might as well have been in China. While she was working her tail off, he disappeared into his office, buried himself in work, and shirked all family responsibilities. By the end of the day, she was seriously miffed. And she laid into him. She slammed his selfish behavior. Criticized his work habits. Told him what a lousy manager he was, and how he was responsible for putting his business in such a sorry state.

In other words, she blasted him for just about everything she could think of, none of which had anything to do with what had really made her angry. Her husband, of course, was totally blindsided. All he'd done was take a few minutes to catch up on work, he pleaded. And for some reason she really seemed to *hate* him.

Sound familiar? When we get angry, we lash out. The longer an issue festers, the angrier we get, and the nastier the fight is likely to be. This woman had every right to be angry. Her husband was doing (or wasn't doing) things that would have annoyed anyone. But rather than addressing those specific issues, she took it global and attacked everything possible.

Deal with the issue.
- Deal with feelings first. It's easy to criticize or judge others for behavior we don't approve of, or hammer them for personal or professional shortcomings. Even when criticism is warranted, it shouldn't come at the expense of what the other person is feeling. Let your partner know that he or she is loved and cared for. That comes first. After that, by all means criticize; but do it gently and with love.

- Use "I" when expressing anger. It's easy to throw around the word "you" ("You make me furious when you do that"). A better approach is to use "I." ("I get angry when you do that.") This makes it clear that you're upset without attacking the other person personally.

- Respond, don't react. Minor squabbles can quickly escalate into full-blown fights when people get angry and blurt out the first hurtful thing that comes to mind. You can defuse almost any situation when you *respond* to the situation rather than immediately *react* to the words or behavior that made you angry. Talk about what makes you angry, but without expressing the anger itself.

- Don't make it personal. Suppose your husband makes a wrong turn when you're on a trip. You could criticize his behavior by saying something like, "Didn't you see the sign back there? Anyone could see it. What's wrong with you?" At that moment, he's unlikely to respond with gratitude. He's probably going to respond with equal anger and sarcasm. Since the event—missing the turn—is the main issue, deal *only* with that. "We missed the turn. Why don't we turn around?"

- If you are angry and boiling, step back, take a deep breath, and *wait* to confront your partner. In the meantime, take a moment to clearly define the issue in your own mind. What's really bothering you? A specific issue? Or something broader?

- Think about a solution that will satisfy you. Maybe all you need is an apology. Maybe you want something to change in the future. Either way, there must be some endpoint that you hope to reach.

4. To be a better man, think like a woman

Personally I feel sorry for the Macho Man, the tough dude who takes no prisoners. He's always in charge. He's a "leader" who takes no flak from anyone—including his partner. This is obviously an exaggeration of a cliché, but many men don't even come close to understanding the power of intimacy. They're so closed off in their hearts that their lives are likely incomplete. These men rarely have satisfying relationships.

For most women, nurturing is the very essence of connectedness and love. They know how important it is to comfort and support, to be there in times of need. Men can learn a lot from women. True intimacy means sharing your vulnerabilities with your partner. Admitting when you're afraid. Talking about what concerns you. Men who share themselves get an equal measure in return. True love is unconditional. Men who know this are willing to share *everything* … because they know they won't be hurt.

A good relationship is always a partnership, not a hierarchy. No one is the boss, nor should they be.

5. Love is much more important than sex
Many men I know—and I'd have to include myself among them—are beggars when it comes to sex. What a shameful commentary on men! There's nothing wrong with wanting sex and asking for sex. There's something very wrong with demanding it. Sex is not a "right." It's about giving, a shared joy that uplifts both partners' spirits. Arguing about sex, or attacking your partner because she (or he) doesn't "perform" the way you want, never works.

My advice, always, is to forget the sex for the time being. Instead, think about being together. Only that. Sexual intimacy has very little to do with just intercourse. It's about being tender and romantic, about passionate touching and talk. A man who truly loves his wife will experience great pleasure in bringing his partner to orgasm whether or not he can have an erection. Women have their share of sexual problems, which I'll discuss in the next chapter. For both men and women, it's worth remembering that sex is just another expression of intimacy. The couples that stay together know this. They'll find other ways to stay close when the sex isn't happening.

6. Relationships always change—so adjust!
It seems like only yesterday that my wife and I were dating, then raising children, then watching them go off to college and starting

their own lives. Time flies! And the rules of the game change every day. With every year and decade, work schedules shift, children need more or less attention, our parents need our help, and on and on. Couples who don't adapt to all of these changes, who see themselves as somehow fixed in time, don't last very long.

A good friend of mine, also a doctor, is married to a woman who chose to stay home and raise her children. Their youngest is now in high school. Like many women who give a lot of their years to raising children, she decided it was time to try something new. A year ago, she went to work for an investment broker, and quickly became one of the company stars. The CEO offered her a very senior position, one with incredible possibilities for personal and financial success. The downside: it would require a move to Atlanta.

Her son didn't want to leave his school. Her husband, a surgeon in private practice, was adamant that he needed her at home. Ripe grounds for conflict, for sure! She was understandably angry. She had supported him for years, she said, and now it was *her* turn. They could have gone to war—and honestly, I'm not sure how long the peace will hold—but for now they've compromised. She rented an apartment in Atlanta, and plans to commute to be with her family every weekend. Her husband, still somewhat resentful, has made it clear he'll never pack up and leave. How will it work out? Who knows? Personally, I have very little sympathy for the husband. He might not want to move, but he'd do fine in another state; and I think she was right. It *is* her turn.

This is a rather big kind of compromise. In daily life, there are scores of smaller ones: whether or not to invest in a new business or move to a smaller house. There's rarely a perfect decision. Couples that stay together know this. They work together to find a middle ground that may not be perfect, but that is a lot better than landing in divorce court.

All changes, big or small, have the potential to bring couples closer together or drive them further apart. The big changes, such as retirement or children leaving home, can dramatically upset a contented equilibrium. I've known a lot of couples who did just fine while raising the kids. Then when the kids were gone and this shared responsibility was past, they realized just how little they had in common. Not every relationship can be saved. But most can be as long as both partners are flexible enough to work together and make the necessary shifts as their circumstances change.

7. Every relationship takes work

It's amazing the things patients let slip when they're in my office. Things like:

- "He does his thing and I do mine."

- "We hardly talk any more, and when we do it always ends in an argument."

- "I know all her warts, and after all these years, they irritate me more than ever."

- "He doesn't even know I exist. At the breakfast table, all I see is the sports page."

- "What other man would look at her? You have got to be kidding."

- "I wish he would have an affair. At least he'd leave me alone."

Whew! Many of these couples have been together for decades … and *that's* the way they feel about each other? Any relationship with that kind of venom needs work. Delivered with a smile or not, words like those are cutting and reflect a huge amount of underlying animosity. In those sorts of relationships, the animosity builds over years. They didn't start out that way, but rather underlying problems festered and bubbled until the two partners drift completely apart—never really seeing one another. This is a prescription for disaster.

Every relationship needs work, no matter how long you've been together. You must constantly work together to ensure that both partners are growing in the same direction. Do whatever it takes to show that you care. Make a date night every week. Plan a vacation together—or even take separate vacations, as long as you come back to the relationship renewed and committed to work. Do things together, like gardening, hiking, politics, whatever. And at least once a day, reaffirm that contract, written or otherwise, that holds you and your partner together. "I love you" are three words that never get dull.

8. Love grows

It's an interesting thing. We tend to think of love and passion as the province of the young, but the opposite seems to be true. Surveys of couples indicate that those in their 50s have a much higher level of love and commitment than those in their 30s. Maybe it's because it takes maturity and seasoning to feel more at ease with ourselves and more comfortable with others. At the same time, couples in their 50s and older tend to have fewer demands on their time. They're less involved with children, for the most part, and have more time for each other.

Everything slows down as we age, sex included. There's more time for foreplay since reaching orgasm takes longer. This prolonged intimacy may be why people in their 60s and older often report being more satisfied with their sex lives than those in their 20s or 30s. And when were you more likely to take the time to enjoy the sunset—when you were in your 20s or in your 50s or 60s? Who better to enjoy it with than someone you truly love?

9. Commitment counts

In her recent book, Dr. Cherie Carter Scott describes the five stages of love. The first stage is *connection*. This is the palpable connection that you feel with someone you're truly attracted to. Then comes *exploration*, the getting-to-know-you phase. This is when you discover how much you have in common, when you realize that romance is hovering in the air. It's also a tricky time, because people in this stage tend to overlook, or dismiss, the things that aren't so good. The third phase, *evaluation*, is when couples start to make the hard decisions: if they're truly compatible, if they think they can live together, if they have similar goals, faiths, and so on. The fourth stage is *building intimacy*. Dr. Scott eloquently defines intimacy as "opening the door and allowing your partner to see the truth of who you are in all dimensions" Finally comes the fifth and most important stage: *commitment.*

The contract of marriage—or, indeed, any long-term relationship— requires a very strong commitment. It's a tough decision to make. People are afraid of getting hurt, and past experiences can hinder them from fully moving forward. Make no mistake: There's no such thing as a sort-of commitment. It's all or nothing. Couples that make this commitment are far more likely to stay together than those who, consciously or not, are always leaving their options open.

Commitment doesn't happen all at once. For some couples, it might occur in months; others might not get there for years. But successful couples invariably take this crucial step.

10. Get help before giving up

I would never argue that a bad marriage is better than divorce, but always seek help before throwing in the towel on a relationship. Many relationships can be salvaged—and can come to thrive—if the partners put enough energy into making it happen. It's almost always a mistake to give up too easily.

A troubled marriage can often be saved by professional intervention with a therapist or marriage counselor. At the very least, timely counseling can help ensure a more respectful separation. A leading psychiatrist, Dr. Harold Koenig, has described in his research couples that, to all appearances, had truly irreconcilable differences. Yet even in those relationships, when the partners shared a strong belief in fidelity and commitment, the marriages could often be saved.

I don't mean to paint too rosy a picture. Some people aren't meant to be together. But ending a marriage is so cataclysmic for all concerned that it only makes sense to try to fit the pieces back together. If you fail, well, at least you'll always know you tried. Counseling takes time. It also requires a near-fanatical commitment on the part of both partners to make things work. Most couples who come through the crucible of therapy intact look back on it as a tremendous opportunity to foster personal growth, gain a deeper knowledge of flaws and personal failings, and, finally, to understand the underlying issues that led the relationship into crisis mode.

Love beyond marriage: lessons of companionship *and* community

When we talk about love, we tend to limit the issue to intimate relationships. Ultimately, the science and research has been limited to intimate relationships as well. I've mentioned that love comes in many forms and any relationship is better than no relationship, but let's take a minute to look a why being in a relationship promotes health.

Perhaps the most obvious benefit of being in a relationship (whether it's a friend or companion) is the loneliness factor. Relationships keep people connected and engaged with life. Studies show that people who spend a lot of time alone and don't have close connections with family or friends have more depression and illness, and die younger, than those with busy social schedules. Socially active people are far more likely to retain their independence throughout their lives. It's critically important to have a life full of love and companionship. This is especially true as we reach our 80s and beyond, when various health problems—and the all-too-frequent deaths of friends and partners—greatly increase our need for emotional support.

When discussing companionship and health, I always end up using the same example: my mother. My mother, Hanid, married my late father at 18 and had a passionate and wonderful marriage. Unfortunately, he suffered a fatal heart attack while she was still relatively young. She remarried soon after he died, and again was lucky enough to enjoy some lovely years. When her second husband passed away, my mother—who has never been called a shrinking violet—was once again thrust back into the dating scene. Eventually she married again. At the time she was in her 70s (and he in his 80s). Naïve Jewish son that I am, I figured that this time would be the charm. Nope. A few years later, my mom booted him out the door.

She still wasn't ready to give up. She threw herself back into the dating world with a vengeance. Pretty soon she was dating two men, one on Tuesdays and Saturdays and another on Wednesdays and Sundays. Just to keep things lively, she soon added a third man, Cecil, into the mix; he was the man who quickly became her true love.

She didn't marry this time; his religious beliefs prohibited him from marrying a divorcée. But this was the relationship she'd been waiting for. The two of them lived across the street from each other, spending time equally at each other's houses. They were together for over ten years and I know that my mother's health was improved by his presence in her life. Unfortunately, Cecil recently passed away at age 99. Although we all knew it was coming, and my mother had tried to prepare herself for his death, it still took an enormous toll. For the first time in over 65 years, my mother no longer has a man in her life. Yes, she has friends and family and loads of people who dote on her regularly. But the loss of her true love was no less powerful. Today, I am worried about her health. Though she has very few physical medical problems, this loss of love is enough to send her downhill. While my mother's endless search for love and companionship provided the quintessential example of how love promotes health, perhaps the latest turn of events—losing love at 85—is an even more powerful account of why we need more love at any age.

My mother's story resonates with me not just as a concerned son, but also as 66-year-old man. For me, and many of my baby boomer friends, losing love after retirement is a serious concern. We may lose love through divorce, illness, relocation, and even death; but the end result will be the same. What would I do if I found myself single again? Could I be as strong as my mother and jump out there again at 70 or 75? Though I cannot even begin to imagine what that would be like, I know that the worst thing to do is give up. Marriage isn't the point. Nor is dating, at least in the traditional sense. But as you age and inevitably lose loved ones, it is critical to fill your life with love *of any kind*.

If you do lose that intimate love of a monogamous relationship, then sometimes the issue of *companionship* morphs into *community*. A strong community of love and support may stand in for a lack of companionship. Remember, love reaches beyond the confines of a one-on-one relationship. Many of us find love through an entire network or community. This may be your church community, college friends, a book club, a golfing group, or whatever else gives you a sense of belonging and connectedness.

For us baby boomers, retirement forces all of us to contemplate seriously this idea of community. Will you relocate? Will you downsize your house? Will you move to a place where you have no pre-existing support base? Will you see your family? All of these questions need attention.

At some point, most of us have had the revelation that our social lives are more limited than they used to be. When you're young, you have built-in social networks: living with your family, going to school, and so on. Once people leave the nest and go out in the world, things start to narrow. How many people socialize with their neighbors? How many even *know* their neighbors? So what does that mean for your community? In the world of Robert Putnam's *Bowling Alone*, will baby boomers find love and connection outside the nuclear family?

A very interesting phenomenon is happening around the world right now: rogue aging baby boomers are redefining community and choosing to build their own intentional communities that fit their needs as aging adults. In Arizona, a group of friends decided to create an intergenerational community of "co-housing," where meals were shared and milestones were celebrated by all. Certainly a more sophisticated "commune" than what we envision from the 1960s, this community was created specifically to foster an increased sense of connectedness and sustainable living.

Though this Arizona community may seem too far out there, we often forget that human beings have always lived in groups. It's only in the last 60 years or so that the *nuclear* family became the norm. In a further narrowing of our social ties, living alone has become more and more common. In the 1950s, fewer than 10% of American adults lived alone. In recent years, that percentage is closer to 25%. Many people prefer living alone, and it's certainly possible for "singletons" to maintain close-knit social groups. But the risk of isolation rises considerably when you live alone, and the effects of isolation on health are profound. As more and more baby boomers reach retirement, especially if they are without an intimate relationship, I am sure that the issue of community will continue to arise. We must strive to foster environments in which people can open themselves up to one another and develop new bonds of love.

So I challenge you to begin today thinking about community, connectedness, and love. There is clearly no prescription or white paper on how to create love in your life, but here are some good ways to start.

Accept love in all its forms. Love of family, love of friends, love of God—it doesn't matter, as long as you love. The more connected you are to the world around you, the less you'll get sick, and the longer you'll live. You'll also have a lot more fun along the way.

Spend time with your children, grandchildren or other relatives. Family is the most powerful form of unconditional love. It is safe, unconditional, supportive, complete.

Get out of the house. I know too many people for whom the very idea of a social evening makes them cringe. Get used to it! Set up dinner invitations. Meet at a nearby restaurant. Check out a gallery opening. Show up at a knitting club. Join a few church committees. Talk to new people, even if your natural instincts are to stand apart.

Always remember that love is the key to longevity: it sustains, nurtures, stabilizes, and reassures. Love exists in many forms; with your spouse or partner it is complete, trusting and hopefully passionate and sexual, with a child pure and unconditional, with a friend comfortable and knowing, and with your community proud, involved, and committed.

CHAPTER 5
MORE (AND BETTER) SEX

I love being 66. All the stereotypes are out the window and life with my Medicare card is only getting better. With each passing year I grow more sensible and at peace with every aspect of my life. I am more understanding, wiser, and—compared with my younger days—no longer obsessed with sex! While this may sound like a less than positive change, it has actually brought me much closer and more in love with my wife. Losing the obsession with sex allowed me to look beyond my own physical yearnings and see my wife as a gorgeous, sexy, and totally irresistible. Sex has changed with each decade—and, I can honestly say, it's better than ever.

If you think sex ends after 60, you're wrong. Plain and simple. For many baby boomers, the sexual revolution of the 1960s was just a precursor to what's ahead. Today's revolution is about redefining sex and aging. The sexiest icons of our youth now have grey hair and grandchildren … but, somehow, they're sexier than ever!

While sex is still a major part of baby boomers' lives, all of us are facing the realities of how sex changes with age. Sex at 60 is not like sex at 35. Frankly, I wouldn't want it to be. Your emotions change, your body changes, and your relationships change as well. But when it comes to mature sex, the bottom line is to do what makes you feel good! Do what works today, not what worked 30 years ago.

The fourth step in Dr. David's Longevity Plan is *more* sex. People who have more sex tend to be happier and healthier than those who don't. While sex is not a major predictor for living a healthy life, it is still an important element for many couples. If you are still interested and inspired to enjoy a healthy sex life, don't let age slow you down. When it comes to sex after 60, it's important to understand how aging affects your sex life and what you can do to keep the spark going.

Sex changes

Recently, I had an interesting discussion with a close colleague who shed some insight into how sex actually improves with age. After 30 years of marriage, he was madly in love with his wife—totally and without reservation. Their relationship was not without problems and the usual conflicts about money (there was always too little) and sex (there was never enough) persisted. But over the years they fought less and appreciated each other more. For them, sex in the Medicare era had never been better … maybe not as frequent, but definitely sexier and more passionate.

We all look back somewhat wistfully at our younger, presumably more sexual, selves. But try to take an honest look through the pleasant haze of memory. Sex at 20 wasn't all that great! Inexperience was like a cold shower. I was constantly nervous, worried about not pleasing my partner. I was too embarrassed to say what I liked or didn't like, and definitely too unsure to ask my partner what she liked. At that age, sex was a harshly judged performance! Only with age and experience did my sexual worries abate. Truthfully, it took me six kids and two marriages to realize that sex was more about sharing pleasures than pleasing myself! It comes as no surprise that 48% of adults over the age of 65 profess to be "very happy" with their sex lives, compared to approximately 25% of adults between the ages of 18 and 31. In a study conducted by the National Council on Aging, 70% of respondents over the age of 65 were happier with their sex lives than they had been in their 40s.

Your attitude toward sex changes with age, and your body changes as well. If you expect to function exactly the same at 60 as at 20, get ready for disappointment. But that doesn't mean it's any less satisfying or complete! To the horror of their children, older couples are still having sex! It may happen less often—but it's just as good.

My conviction that sex gets better with age is something of a hard sell. In our image-obsessed culture, we're inundated with media messages that tell us that "sexy" and "young" are synonymous. If you have gray hair, wrinkles, and a less-than-perfect body, sex is unattainable, unsatisfying, and possibly even unappetizing. But the vast amounts of sexuality research that has been conducted in the last few decades, along with the zesty stories I hear from my less-inhibited patients, suggest something quite different. Yes, sex changes. For some people, it might change for the worse. But for many others, sex gets, well, sexier, with advancing age.

Sex after 60: the data

Despite my fervent case that sex gets better with age, many of my middle-aged friends still buy into the stereotypes of sex and aging. They all ask the same questions: Is it all going to be downhill from here? Will I ever be truly "horny" again? Will the spark disappear completely? Are we condemned to struggle with infrequent or un-satisfying sex? Beyond my own anecdotes, even research suggests that the answer is no.

It's time to abandon the notion that sex ends with old age! In August 2007, the *New England Journal of Medicine* published select results from of a large study conducted at the University of Chicago. In the University of Chicago's National Social Life, Health and Aging Project, researchers surveyed 1500 men and 1440 women ranging in age from 57 to 85 years. When it came to sex, their findings may seem surprising.

Greater than 60% of the entire group maintained that sexuality remained an important part of their life. Not surprisingly, sex remained more important to men than to women. Seventy-three percent of individuals between 57 and 64 years were sexually active with at least one partner. Between the ages of 64 and 74, the percentage dropped to 57%, and after the age of 75 it dropped again to 23%. Overall, women were less likely to be sexually active than men. But the women were also significantly less likely to be in a marital or intimate relationship. This difference increased dramatically with advancing age.

At any given age, health and sexuality were clearly linked. Those with poor health had less sex. Sexual dysfunction or the presence of a significant illness (heart attack, back pain, stroke) was the most likely explanation for a decline in sexual activity. Even among those who remained sexually active, over half reported a sexual problem.

Unfortunately, only 38% of men and 22% of women had ever discussed sexuality or sexual problems with a physician.

The Longevity Factor
Beyond its feel-good aspects, sex actually improves your quality of life. Studies even show there is a correlation between sexual activity and longevity.

A study reported in the *British Medical Journal* found that men who had frequent orgasms—more than two a week—were 50% less likely to die than those who had orgasms less than once a month. Men who had sex twice a week were three times less likely to have a heart attack than those who had sex less than once a month!

Incidentally, what's good for the gander appears to be equally beneficial for the goose, but with a twist. While sexual frequency is directly linked to longevity in men, sexual satisfaction is much more important for women. Researchers at Duke University's Center on Aging have found that the enjoyment of sex is a powerful predictor of reduced mortality. In other words, women who enjoy sex live longer, regardless of how often they have it. Conversely, women who are dissatisfied with their sex lives are more likely to have heart attacks than those who are sexually satisfied.

Researchers cannot adequately explain why sex appears to be protective. The question tends to get a little murky. Married men are more likely to have frequent sex than single men, and we know that married men live longer than those who are single, widowed, or divorced. So it's possible that marriage, rather than sex, causes these men to live longer. On the other hand, perhaps sex stimulates physical changes in the body that promote long-term health. Sex may reduce stress, which in turn reduces health risks. In the end, it's likely that sex is a symptom of a good relationship rather than a cause. Healthy, loving relationships promote longevity.

Sex and the aging body
There's no getting around it, sex changes as your body changes. Certain parts just don't seem to work as well as they used to—I hate

to say it, but it's only natural. Just like you can't sprint up the stairs as fast as you used to, you may not be able to go at it in bed with as much vigor and stamina as years past. Without doubt, arousal takes longer with age. But there is no reason for these natural, age-related changes to dampen or inhibit your ability to have sex or be a great lover.

Let's look at what happens to your body during sexual arousal and activity.

First, all arousal starts in the brain. This is the key to launching a physiological chain reaction to fuel any sexual encounter. When the brain is stimulated, it sends chemical signals—in the forms of *neuropeptide Y, vasointestinal polypeptide*, and *nitric oxide*—through the central nervous system. The chemical rush creates the surge of arousal and allows subsequent sexual activity. In men, these signals are simultaneously sent to the penis and prostate gland, promoting erection; in women, the signals go to the clitoris, vagina, and uterus, causing relaxation and lubrication.

Hormones also play a key role in arousal. Estrogen, for example, promotes vaginal muscle tone and lubrication. Lubrication does more than make sex comfortable, it also makes the vagina somewhat acidic and less hospitable to yeast and other infections. Not just a "male hormone," testosterone plays a role in women's sexual health as well.

Ultimately, there are three main components that must be present in a healthy sexual experience: your brain, your hormones, and healthy pathways for chemical signals to affect your blood and tissues. Problems in any of these areas can result in reduced sex drive, impotence, loss of lubrication, and so on.

For men, the height of sexual functioning occurs around age 18. Young men can often have multiple erections and orgasms on any given night, and they can repeat the performance night after night. Nature's irony, of course, is that men of this age are unlikely to have steady relationships or the necessary time or privacy in which to indulge.

After age 18, a man's sexual functioning slowly declines. With time, it becomes more difficult to get an erection, and erections are less firm. It takes longer to achieve orgasm and even more time to recover and reach climax again. All of these factors contribute to the fact that by age 50 most men are having about half as much sex as they did in their younger years.

While physical changes can affect the logistics of sex, they have little effect on a man's ability to enjoy a varied and active sex life. It may take more effort, more foreplay, and more touching to achieve that erection, but so what? It's time well spent! Plus, there's a happy trade-off. Older men are generally "slower on the trigger." It takes them longer to get erect, but once they have an erection they're able to make it last longer. With less regular erections, many older men learn more creative ways to induce those sexual feelings. And since women typically require more time to achieve orgasm, this "delay" often makes sex more satisfying for both parties.

Women reach their sexual peaks much later than men, usually between the ages of 35 and 40. However, as women reach menopause and beyond, gradual declines in estrogen and progesterone occur. When estrogen levels decline at menopause, the loss of lubrication can make sex less comfortable. In addition, lower levels of estrogen can reduce libido and the ability to have orgasms. Menopausal declines in testosterone can cause a decline in libido. These hormonal changes lead to thinning of the lining of the vagina that can cause dryness and a reduced ability to lubricate when aroused. This can lead to difficulties with penetration and painful sex.

In addition to decreased libido and slower arousal, women's ability to climax during sex also decreases with age. Between the ages of 40 and 50, 33% of women report that they always have an orgasm with their partner. On the other hand, between the ages of 50 and 60, the percentage drops to 26%. Interestingly, despite the diminishing frequency of orgasms, older women are more satisfied with their sex lives than are their younger counterparts. It's easy to presume that the emotional components of mature sex bring as much, or more, satisfaction than the orgasmic fireworks of a horny twenty-something. Studies show that 40% of women over age 50 feel that they're better lovers than they were when they were younger.

Let's talk about sex

For many adults, sex is an important part of a healthy relationship. Sadly, sexual problems can undermine even the most healthy and committed relationship. Because it can play such a critical role, every physician should discuss it with his or her patients. Unfortunately, sex is a difficult subject for everyone to discuss … doctors and patients alike.

For me, learning to discuss and understand the realities of mature sex was a process. I still remember the first patient who forced me to talk about sex and aging. She came to me because her other doctor told her to "not expect much." Though I felt uncomfortable and awkward, I had to help this woman—who could have been my mother—have better sex! Believe me, for a young physician, it was a steep learning curve.

This 78-year-old widow loved sex! She maintained an active dating life and went dancing three nights a week. At first glance, it seemed she was enjoying sex more than ever. Unfortunately, at her age, she started to develop some of the more difficult challenges of an aging body. Simply put, vaginal dryness was slowing her down. Intercourse was painful and "oral sex only goes so far," she complained.

As she was recounting her various sexual problems, I was shocked by her candor. She so readily complained and, what's more, she knew that it could be fixed. I had to admit it: this woman knew more about sex and aging than I did. She opened my eyes, for sure.

Fortunately for both of us, treatment was easy. I sent her away with some estrogen cream and a water-based lubricant, and she was good to go. The cream restores vaginal strength, while the lubricant eases the way. She came back a month later with a grin on her face and said proudly, "three times a week!" She's now pushing 90, and continues to have sex once or twice a week. She usually has orgasms and has to take it easy on her partner!

Today I ask my patients about sex for two main reasons. First, maintaining a healthy sex life is a powerful predictor of long-term health. Second, changes in sexual activity may be a sign of other potentially serious problems. If my patients aren't having sex, or there have been changes in their usual sexual activities, I want to know about it. Not surprisingly, most of my patients are reluctant to talk about sex. We'll usually spend half an hour discussing whatever health problem brought them in the door, then, when they're about ready to leave, they'll spring something like "do you think Viagra will help me?" Surprise, surprise. The real reason they came in arises and, without fail, we sit back down and discuss what's going on behind closed doors.

For physicians assessing sexual problems, it's important to evaluate both partners. You have to know the whole story. Here is a good example. When I was much younger and less experienced, I saw a patient who complained of erectile dysfunction. In those days there were no medications to treat the problem, so I prescribed a vacuum tumescence device (also known as a "penis pump"). This involves putting a tube over the penis and creating a vacuum that causes the penis to become erect. A band is then placed over the base of the penis to maintain the erection. The patient was delighted that it worked so well! Well, a few days later his very irate wife called me on the phone complaining that I had ruined her life. This couple had not had sex in five years, and nor had they been very intimate. Suddenly her husband walks into the bedroom with a large erection and tells her he's "ready." She was furious—and it was all my fault!

If you are still interested in maintaining a health sex life, do not ignore *any* sexual issues! Don't give up and assume it's a "natural" part of aging. Don't be embarrassed: just talk to a doctor. The vast majority of sex problems can be resolved, usually without enormous investments in time or energy.

Where's the spark?

If the spark is missing (and you want it back) there are two distinct components to address. Physical problems can be corrected rather easily, while emotional problems may be more difficult. Remember, sex is a *couple's* issues. Both people must be willing to fix the problem. Though this sounds obvious, many people feel to uncomfortable talking about sex with their partners, choosing rather to take the burden on themselves and solve the problem alone.

Ignoring sexual concerns or refusing to talk candidly with your spouse can cause a serious rift in the relationship. Even after decades of marriage, couples can drift apart, rarely touching, kissing, or sharing intimacy. This lack of connectedness is harmful to your relationship and your health. A patient once told me that she was reluctant to touch, kiss, or cuddle her husband because of his erectile dysfunction. She feared that he would view her kisses as a sexual overture and become uncomfortable, ashamed, or embarrassed. So they slept on opposite sides of their king-sized bed and both husband and wife felt sad and unfulfilled. There was so much miscommunication between them. While she was concerned about hurting his feelings, he thought she no longer found him attractive. All it took was a little candor and discussion, and this couple virtually transformed. Communication is the key to a healthy sex life.

When it comes to trouble in the bedroom, older adults typically fall into one of three main categories: doesn't want to have sex at all, wants to have sex but can't get going, and can start having sex but never achieves orgasm.

No sex, no problem

A 2006 study in the journal *Menopause* found that nearly a third of partnered women between 50 and 70 have little or no sex drive. Reduced libido is by far the most common cause of sexual dysfunction in women. However, for both men and women, reduced libido is rarely just a plumbing issue.

For women especially, good sex is strongly associated with an intimate and healthy relationship. If the love is lost, or missing, sex can naturally become difficult. From overt marital problems like infidelity and fighting to seemingly benign problems like boredom and a sense of complacency, any issue that affects the relationship will likely affect the bedroom. Remember, love is the best sexual enhancer you will ever find. And there are ways to rekindle a loving relationship.

You can still feel the love without wanting to have sex. For both men and women, there are many other physical causes of reduced libido. Declines in hormone levels can definitely play a role, especially for women who experience declines in estrogen and testosterone after menopause. For some women, prescribing hormone replacement therapy containing small amounts of testosterone can dramatically improve libido. Some doctors are also prescribing Viagra for women. Though not approved for improving a woman's sex drive, some people do experience good results.

It's considerably less common for men to experience reduced libido due to hormone loss. Whenever a man who complains of problems with libido, I will first measure testosterone levels. If the levels are found to be very low, replacement of testosterone using an injection, cream, or a patch can be very helpful in returning libido to normal.

Illnesses and medications can also have a huge effect on your sex drive. Research has shown that as many as 40% of women who have had breast cancer develop sexual dysfunction. The emotional impact of coping with illness combined with the potential for side effects of various medications can virtually halt a person's willingness for sex. From cancer and heart disease to depression and hypertension, any medical conditions should definitely be addressed in the quest to add a little spice in the bedroom.

Because of the complex nature of sexual interest, arousal, and performance, it's not surprising that many drugs, especially those with multiple actions in the body, might cause trouble. Take a complete list of all medications—both over-the-counter and prescription—to your physician to identify any sexual side effects. With the help of a pharmacist, your physician should look at each and every drug to see if it might be causing problems. If they identify a potential problem, you may be able to switch to an alternative medication or change dosages.

Here is a wonderful example of a true success story. One of my patients, a handsome, 67-year-old man, is married to one of the most exciting and voluptuous women I've ever met. After years of marriage, his sex life had dwindled. He was too tired, uninterested, and simply did not want to have sex. There didn't seem to be anything wrong with him that would explain the intense fatigue and disinterest.

After peeling back the layers of this patient's problem, he ultimately admitted that he was completely impotent. He had tried Viagra, but it didn't help. He was so depressed and ashamed about the problem that he had given up on sex all together.

Determined to help this man, I took a look at his list of medications. It turned out he was taking *gemfibrozil*, an older cholesterol-lowering drug that causes impotence in about 12% of men who take it. Even if he needed help lowering cholesterol (blood tests later revealed that he did not), this was not the right drug for him.

I told him to quit taking it. Bingo. His depression ceased, the fatigue lifted, and the next time I saw him, he gave a wink and a smile. The loss of libido was a symptom of a more complex issue – but easily treatable nonetheless.

The spirit says "yes" but the body won't cooperate

Many older adults find themselves emotionally willing to have sex, but just can't seem to get aroused. Or, if they do get going, sex is difficult, painful, or achieving an orgasm may be a challenge.

When it comes to most **arousal disorders**, the common cause is lack of use. For your sexual health, the mantra may be "use it or lose it." This is an additional cause of erectile dysfunction in men. For women, it can present with physical difficulties. The vagina may remain dry and sex will definitely be painful. After one or two painful experiences, it's easy to see how it's difficult to get aroused!

Really work on increasing sexual activity. Men who can have erections should masturbate more, either alone or with their partner. This also applies to women for whom a sexual toy may work very well. Always use a water-based lubricant. Women with dryness and painful sex should discuss the problem with their doctor. Estrogen creams may be appropriate.

Ultimately, whenever combating issues of pain or physical limitations, it's vital that both people make a commitment to have enjoyable sexual encounters—with or without penetration. Foreplay should last as long as possible. Experiment with different positions, adult movies, or role-playing. You never know what might get you going!

Then, there are those people who have no problem initiating sex, but have **difficulty achieving orgasm.** As with everything in health, addressing this medical issue often requires more than just a prescription. The "lifestyle" element of this health concern may mean changing the way you have sex. Good sex does not have to be a mind-blowing, multi-orgasmic experience every time! Orgasms should be seen as a good dessert after a very satisfying meal—you could do without it and still be happy.

Once again, the key is to maximize stimulation and minimize inhibition. Many women are simply much too passive in this regard. Don't wait for your partner to do the right thing. You have to take care of yourself. If this means indulging with a vibrator for half an hour before making love, go for it. You might benefit from Kegel exercises, where you alternately squeeze and relax the pelvic muscles repeating this frequently throughout the day. For some women, Kegels can help promote orgasm. For men, more stimulation may be needed, either through masturbation or oral sex.

The little blue pill

It would be impossible to discuss sex after 60 without mentioning Viagra, the little blue pill that revolutionized mature sex forever. With its massive marketing campaigns and enticing effects, Viagra has literally changed the lives of millions of adult men. Studies show that erectile dysfunction affects 18 million American men, with over 50% of adults 70 years and older experiencing mild to severe problems. Loss of libido, difficulty with arousal, and problems with orgasm can all be symptoms of erectile dysfunction. However, with the advent of Viagra—and its second-generations cousins Levitra and Cialis—most men now turn to pills for the quick fix solution. Based on the results from AARP's Sexuality at Midlife study conducted in 1999 and again in 2004, the number of men who had tried these drugs had doubled, from 10% to over 20%.

But why are so many men affected by erectile dysfunction? In general, there are three main factors:

- **Neurological problems** For an erection to occur you must first send a message from the brain to the penis to become erect. This involves certain hormones and also requires that there be no interruption in the nerve supply to the penis. Any problem with the brain, the spinal cord, or the small nerves entering the penis can lead to erectile dysfunction. Common neurological causes of erectile dysfunction include, strokes, damage to the spinal cord caused by injury and disorders of the back. In addition, damage to nerves that go to the penis also leads to erectile dysfunction. This can be caused by diabetes, alcohol abuse, or surgery to the prostate that may have damaged the nerve supply to the penis.

- **Vascular disease** Once the message from the brain reaches the penis, the muscles in the body of the penis relax and it becomes engorged with blood, which leads to an erection. If the blood supply to the penis is impaired, an erection will not occur. The major cause is *atherosclerosis* or blockages of the arteries. Just like cholesterol can block the coronary artery, so too can it block the penile artery, leading to erectile dysfunction.

- **Psychogenic.** The brain plays a powerful role in sex: if you're stressed, worried, anxious, or depressed, it will certainly affect your abilities. This is especially true with erectile dysfunction. Some men worry so much about their ability to perform, that they psych themselves out of it! Nearly every man on the planet has experienced this problem - especially those with physical problems. If it happens more than once, it can lead to a very uncomfortable cycle. A man who fails to get an erection will worry more the next time. The worry makes him less likely to succeed, which will lead to even more worry. And so on.

If you or your partner experience erectile dysfunction, don't jump to the quick-fix pill right out of the gates! Erectile dysfunction is a treatable medical condition, but a good course of therapy should always begin with counseling. As with every element of health in the bedroom, erectile dysfunction is a couple's issue—not just the man's.

First, erectile dysfunction should not keep you from having an intimate, connected relationship with your partner. Kiss, cuddle, and caress each other. You never know where it might lead. By taking the emphasis away from penetration and orgasm, you'll likely remove many of the mental and emotional barriers associated with ED.

Second, you must understand the underlying cause of erectile dysfunction. Any health condition should be treated and lifestyle counseling should accompany any medical therapy. Remember that physical health and sexual health go hand-in-hand; if you eat well, exercise, and control any medical condition, issues in the bedroom may disappear.

Finally, if both partners understand how sex changes with age and all medical conditions have been addressed, then it's time to consider a medication like Viagra, Cialis, or Levitra. Ultimately, there is little difference between any of these drugs. Viagra and Levitra are very similar. Cialis has a longer half-life and lasts for 36 hours. They work best in younger men, where the problem is more likely related to psychological issues, drugs, or alcohol. In older men, these medications are most successful for those who are able to develop but not sustain an erection.

Most men who take Viagra don't experience serious side effects. Past studies had shown that these medications had negative effects on the heart, but except for those taking medications, this doesn't seem to actually be the case. A recent study in the *Journal of the American Medical Association* found that drugs to treat erectile dysfunction appeared to be safe even in those with relatively severe coronary artery disease.

The older you are and the worse the underlying physical problems, the lower your likelihood for success with erectile dysfunction drugs. Ask your doctor if you'd benefit from injections of prostaglandin or *papaverine* into the penis. While it sounds painful and totally unsexy, the needles are so small that most men hardly feel them and the drugs product strong, long-lasting erections.

Two other options are worth mentioning. The "penis pump" literally sucks blood into the penis. Once an erection occurs, a small rubber band is placed around the base of the penis to maintain the erection. The mechanical approach is off-putting to some men, but the machines do work quite well. If all else fails, your doctor may recommend surgery to implant an inflatable device inside the penis. When a man is ready for sex, all he has to do is press a pump implanted in the groin and an erection springs to life. Men are advised to think long and hard before having the surgery, however. It destroys a man's natural ability to have an erection, so it's only recommended for those who can't be helped in any other way.

Seven steps to rekindle the spark

When it comes down to it, sex is not the most important element of living a healthy, happy and passionate life. If sex is not important to you and your partner, that's okay. But for millions of older adults the bedroom is still a wild and crazy place. Once you understand your body, your partner's body, and the many ways that aging can affect sex, then you're ready to throw the stereotypes away and launch a new sexual revolution—one in which grey is in, wrinkles are sexy, and experience trumps it all.

Next time you want to add a little spice to the bedroom, try these seven steps:

1. Address the physical

The first thing any couple needs to do when addressing sexual problems is **see a doctor.** A doctor can rule out—or address—any physical problems. Sexual dysfunction can occur in both men *and* women. Thanks to Viagra, Cialis and Levitra, the nation is all too aware of erectile dysfunction and impotence. Unfortunately, the female concerns have been largely ignored. Without a "pink" Viagra to shed light on the situation, many women are left feeling that sexual problems—whether lack of interest or pain—are unavoidable. It's not true! This is where a doctor can really help. Get all the physical issues out of the way and then the work in bedroom can really begin.

2. Adjust your attitude

Sex is not always going to be a multi-orgasmic, rock-your-world experience. You have got to let go of your expectations. Remember, sex after 60 is not going to be the same as sex at 35! If you expect it to be, you're destined for failure. Stop living in the past and fantasizing about what sex "used to be" or "should be like." I promise, the past is nowhere near as sexy as the present. So rekindling the spark of any relationship begins in the mind, in the attitudes and expectations of both partners. Start your sexual relationship anew, on a completely blank slate. Do what feels good to you now and be happy with that.

3. Communicate

Communication is the key to a healthy relationship—and, therefore, a healthy sex life. If you have something on your mind, share it with your partner. Otherwise it's bound to come up in the bedroom. For married couples, years of emotional baggage can virtually turn the lights off any libido whatsoever. So it's imperative that you develop a healthy relationship outside of the bedroom. Once you've got the emotional issues resolved, then it's time to talk about the nuts and bolts of sex. Don't be embarrassed to talk about it! If you want more sex, less sex, more touching, less touching—whatever it is, it's time to talk about it. Get it out in the open and you'll be amazed what can happen.

4. Be bold in the bedroom – experiment!

Experimentation is not left for the young! Open your mind to the many fun, exciting, and sexy ways to spice up your sex life. Read some books about it. Rent an erotic movie. Buy a sex toy. Role-play.

Try new positions. Experiment with your fantasies and play them out! Do whatever it takes to cultivate your sexy side—it's in there. Remember, problems is bed have little to do with the mechanics of aging. Lack of creativity will get you every time. So, take it upon yourself to try something new.

5. Create a calendar – for sex.

Nearly every sex therapist will tell you to schedule your time for sex. Though it's the opposite of spontaneous, setting aside time for sex is a great way to get you going. Don't forget the "use it or lose it" mantra. The more regular sex you have, the easier it will be to maintain it. Also by scheduling a time for sex, you and your partner can spend all that lead-up time preparing for the excitement in the bedroom!

6. Be proactive

If you know you're going to have sex, be proactive about taking care of your body and easing any physical pains you might have. Keep water-based lubricant on hand. If you have aches or pains, try taking a pain reliever 30 minutes before. Also, Sue Johanson from the television show "Talk Sex" suggests taking a hot, sensual bath to warm up your joints and muscles. Alternately, she recommends having sex in a chair, which can be easier on your body.

7. Stay healthy

A healthy person is going to have better sex; plain and simple. Be sure to exercise! It will not only build your stamina and endurance, it will also boost your energy. Eat healthy foods. Who wants to have sex after a meal of fried chicken, mashed potatoes and a chocolate cake? You'll be too full for sex! Put food in your body that will give you energy, not take it away. Follow the tenets of this book and you'll not only have a healthier body and mind, but better sex as well.

CHAPTER 6
EMBRACE MORE FAITH

Personally, my road to faith has been circuitous. Perhaps like many baby boomers, I grew up in a traditionally religious family, strayed from organized religion for the bulk of my early adult years, and only returned to spirituality in midlife. As a child, religion was a mandate: a culture and tradition with very clear rules, guidelines, and structures. My image of spirituality was naïve and limited to the actual process of going to worship, setting aside one day of the week for the obligatory prayer and social gatherings. So, as a young adult, it was easy for me to stray. I did not really place a huge value on the tenets of "being religious." Prayer was no more than reading words on a page.

But as I matured as a person—and as a physician—I began to understand that spirituality was much more than a trip to the syna-gogue. Spirituality is a state of being, a way of looking at the world, and a compass for navigating life. As I launched my own personal journey to faith, I also began to discover the indelible link between faith and health. By being more faithful, I was also being healthier.

Just like religion is not as simple as going to a church or mosque, the healthful power of faith is not as simple as merely identifying as a Christian, Jew, Hindu … or anything else. Faith's healing nature lies in the *process* of being spiritual. It is in your actions, your feelings, your words, and your relationships that faith—and the state of being spiritual—can truly impact your health. As a whole, faith clearly affects your health. But specifically the most compelling motivation to be faithful (and healthy) lies with prayer.

The fifth step of Dr. David's Longevity Plan is to have *more* faith and (more specifically) *more* prayer. By embracing your faith and integrating honest, thoughtful prayer into your daily life, you can actually lengthen your life expectancy, reduce risk of ill-ness, and promote your body's own healing nature.

This chapter is divided into two main parts. First we'll discuss the relationship between faith and health in general. Then we'll dive into prayer specifically and discuss *how* believers and non-believers alike can learn to pray.

Before we get started, I must admit that I have come to my own realizations on faith through two distinct means: 1) Scientific research and 2) Personal experience. The culmination of these two processes has allowed me to embrace my faith fully and completely. It has, however, been a long road. So, wherever you are on your personal journey to faith or spirituality, I implore you open yourself to new ideas and thoughts. Throughout this chapter I'll highlight the scientific data to support the relationship between faith, health, and prayer—as well as decidedly less scientific anecdotes. Whether you find solace in the science or the stories, it doesn't matter. This step to living a healthier, more passionate life is appropriate to anyone ... with or without a religious preference.

Faith and health – a scientific perspective

A few decades ago, most reputable physicians and scientists, regardless of their personal beliefs, left contemplating the relationship between faith and health to the fringes of social research. It didn't matter that hundreds of thousands of Americans would cite faith as a major factor for healing! As far a traditional science was concerned, medicine and faith were considered inviolate spheres — useful separately, worse than useless when together.

Today, everything has changed. Nearly every major health organization recognizes faith as a hugely important component of health – not just as a social phenomenon, but as an important predictor of disease prevention, recovery, and even mortality. What's more, those same organizations are funding intense studies and projects to examine every aspect of faith, spirituality, and religion.

Some of the best research has come out of the Center for Spirituality, Theology and Health, based in the Center for Aging at Duke University. Researchers there have concluded that people who believe in a higher power (*any* higher power) are healthier than those who don't. They live longer. They're less likely to develop common illnesses. They cope with illness better, and they have better and faster recovery rates. What was once mere speculation is now supported by clear data.

The idea that belief in a higher power directly relates to your health is a startling concept, particularly for non-believers. Ultimately, the scientific community, including doctors who are religious themselves, don't know what to make of it. But consider this: Of the roughly 125 medical schools in the United States, more than half now offer courses in spirituality and prayer. Academic researchers have published hundreds of studies looking at prayer and health, about two-thirds of which have shown positive results—in patients with cardiovascular disease, diabetes, and infection with HIV, to name just a few. Epidemiological research (in which scientists examine large populations to identify the differences between people who get sick and those who don't) has consistently shown that faith is strongly protective; people who pray or attend church get sick less often, recover more quickly when they do get sick, and live longer. More impressive, many double-blind, placebo-controlled studies— the gold standards for scientific research—have shown **people who pray or believe in a higher power are consistently healthier**.

The impact of faith and health has been examined from nearly every aspect of the medical profession – and the results have touched on nearly every major illness.

Take these examples:

Heart Disease:
Thomas Oxman, M.D., a psychiatrist at Dartmouth Medical School, took a look at 232 patients 55 years and older who were undergoing open-heart surgery. He found that those of strong faith who attended services regularly and were active in their congregations had a 14-fold lower mortality rate during the six months after surgery than those without the same degree of religious commitment. A 14-fold difference! A drug company would go bananas for results like that.

Alzheimer's Disease:
A study at Duke University looked at about 1,700 older adults and found that those who attended weekly services were much more likely to have lower levels of interleukin-6, a protein that may be involved in a variety of age-related diseases, including Alzheimer's disease and osteoporosis.

Cancer:
A very large study that involved 30,000 clergy found that they had a longer life expectancy and a significantly lower risk of lung, gastro-intestinal, and bladder cancer than people in the general popula-tion. Other studies have found that conservative Protestants have lower cancer rates than those of more liberal faiths. (Mormons have the lowest cancer rates.) People who believe in God or some other Higher Power tend to have fewer side effects from chemotherapy. They also recover from infections more quickly.

Hospitalization:
Some of the most compelling research on the ever-shrinking bound-ary between medicine and faith has been conducted by Harold G. Koenig, M.D., professor of psychiatry and behavioral sciences and as-sociate professor of medicine at Duke University School of Medicine. Co-director of the Center for Spirituality, Theology and Health, and author of *The Handbook of Religion and Health*, he has reported that people who attended weekly services were 43 percent less likely to have been hospitalized in the previous year than non-churchgoers. When they were hospitalized (for whatever reason), they spent an average of 14 fewer days in the hospital than non-attenders.

In the spirit of full disclosure, there are many critics of this sort of research. It is particularly difficult to separate the many differ-ent elements of religion. How do social factors come into play? Do socio-economic conditions make a difference? How much of it is simply a placebo effect? Many of these claims are totally valid. Faith, religion, and spirituality are very complex components of both life and health. However, for me, the evidence is compelling enough that it warrants discussion.

Forget the science (for a moment)

Forget the science for a moment. Let me tell a quick story about a rather remarkable couple, Pat and Willard Walker. I met them some years ago, and their personal story, while admittedly anecdotal, gives a wonderful sense of the restorative power of faith. I don't mean faith just in the religious sense, but also in the sense of community, the notion that we all have an obligation to make the world a better place.

Willard was one of the Wal-Mart pioneers. He worked with Sam Walton almost from the beginning, and became incredibly rich as the years went by. Unlike many self-made millionaires, the Walkers didn't see themselves as part of a privileged elite. They fervently believed that it was their obligation to use their wealth to help others less fortunate. So much so that these home-grown philanthropists gave a higher proportion of their income to good causes than virtually anyone else in Arkansas.

I met them because they gave generously to establish the Arkansas Cancer Research Center at the University of Arkansas. They also established a Memory Disorders Center at the Institute on Aging, where I used to work. Willard, I was to discover, had been through some serious health challenges. He developed a rather serious cancer, for which he was treated at the cancer center he helped establish. After the first course of chemotherapy, he had a remission that lasted 10 years. That doesn't happen very often. A decade later, though, the cancer came back in an even more dangerous form. Despite little hope of success, he beat the odds. The tumor disappeared after one course of treatment, and never came back.

Soon after that, Willard developed memory loss due to Alzheimer's disease. Once again, he was in the right place at the right time. A new medication, Tacrine, had just been approved to help improve memory in patients with Alzheimer's. The drug was quite a breakthrough, but hardly perfect. Relatively few of my patients could actually take it due to some nasty side effects. Willard, with his usual luck, had no side effects at all. His memory stayed reasonably good, and for the next 10 years he stayed active. At about that time, the Alzheimer's really picked up steam. Willard died a few year later from heart failure — a disease that his cardiologist had predicted would kill him seven years earlier than it did.

This litany of health problems probably makes Willard's life seem anything but blessed. But we *all* experience health problems as we get older. Willard was fairly typical in that sense, but atypical in that he beat just about every statistical rule in the books. His wife, Pat, also had a few near-miraculous recoveries of her own along the way. Today, at 90, she's in perfect health, lives a complete and full life, and always has a kind word for everyone.

What struck me most about the Walkers, apart from their uncanny ability to prove their doctors wrong, was their profound faith. It infused every part of their lives. These were two people who walked the walk (and didn't do too much talking!). They gave thanks for their blessings every day. They lived with humility and gratitude. Rich almost beyond comprehension, they stayed in the modest, single-level home that they'd lived in for decades. They often said, with a sincerity that was almost breathtaking, how grateful they were for the opportunity to help others.

When I met Pat and Willard, I was not particularly swayed one way or the other on the faith debate. Perhaps this had to do with where I was in my own spiritual path. Perhaps it was because I had not taken the time to really dive into my patients' personal lives before I met them. But, whatever it was, knowing Pat and Willard and seeing how their faith impacted their outlook really pushed me to ask, "Did their faith keep them going?" In the face of serious health problems and major challenges, what role—if any—did their robust belief in God play?

Ultimately, as I contemplate Pat and Willard's life, it's easy to see how their faith offered a guiding force behind every element of their lives. They took care of themselves, surrounded themselves with good friends, and worked closely within their community. They were humble and giving, kind and *forgiving*. They did not harbor resentment toward life—or toward their illnesses. They believed in God and went to church regularly. They prayed and sought God's assistance.

Did they live as fully and healthfully as they did solely because of their religious beliefs? Did they defy the odds and escape death just because of God? I doubt it. But in the end it was their faith that gave them the internal strength to resist just about everything Nature threw their way. They were not just "church-goers," they lived and breathed Christianity.

The power of prayer

One day, while perusing the Internet for interesting health material, I came upon an eye-popping statement that really grabbed my attention ... and challenged the way I thought about health. Here's what it said:

*[It] seems to me to be reprehensible malpractice not to recommend prayer when it is so simple, effective, inexpensive and **proven to be effective**.*

Prayer *proven* to be effective? I wouldn't have given this a second look if it showed up on the website of a faith-based organization, or if it were merely the personal musings of one of the million bloggers out there. But the author, Joseph Mercola, M.D., is a respected physician in the natural-health community. He isn't known for buying into every half-baked theory that comes along. The fact that a truly respected physician was stepping out in the realm of "religious healing" signifies a huge shift in the medical community. The idea that prayer is *proven* to be an effective means of health promotion was one of the first real ways in which health researchers and scientists began to question the link between faith and health.

For those who believe that a Higher Power directly intervenes in worldly affairs, it doesn't require a mental stretch to believe that prayer has salubrious effects. People have likely sought other-worldly help to cure illness for thousands of years. The 21st century is no different. On the popular interfaith website Beliefnet, over three-quarters of the 35,000 online prayer circles are health-related. Tens of thousands of people get online every day to pray for someone's health—their own health, a friend's, a relative's, or even a stranger's.

Quite a few studies over the years suggest that the nature of energy is much more complex than anything you learned in 10th-grade physics. It seems possible that human consciousness can affect energy in ways that simply can't be explained. I recently came across an intriguing experiment done by a Japanese researcher, who, using magnetic resonance technology, found that the molecular arrangements of water can literally be altered by thoughts of love and gratitude. He started out with a water sample taken from a polluted river. A picture of the water looked muddy and lacked a clear crystalline structure. Then he had a temple priest pray to the polluted water. The next picture showed a clear, lovely crystalline structure.

Okay, this is pretty esoteric stuff. I'm not prepared to say that the human thoughts truly have the power to change the physical world. But I can say—and the research backs this up—that people who pray (or meditate) for better health can see positive results. Not every time and for every condition, but often enough that it can't be ascribed to chance. I don't know how it works. I certainly can't say *why* it works. But enough studies have shown positive results that you would have to be completely closed-minded to dismiss this as mere superstition or wishful thinking

Prayer and health: the data
Much research has been done on what is known as "intercessory" prayer. This is when people are prayed for by others rather than praying for themselves. Most scientists have wisely chosen to focus on intercessory prayer rather than personal, "petitionary" prayer. Someone who prays for himself presumably believes in God. He also believes that God may reach out in some fashion and make him better. These and other positive thoughts that accompany petitionary prayer will undoubtedly make him feel better, whether or not the prayer had any actual, measurable effects. In other words, there will be a strong placebo effect. With intercessory prayer, however, it's possible to design studies in which the person being

prayed for doesn't even know it. If he or she shows improvement, then an explanation other than the placebo effect has to be considered.

There have been multiple studies in the last several years examining the role of intercessory prayer on health and recovery and the results have been varied. As you might expect, this has been somewhat of a contentious issue, with scientists, physicians, and researchers on both sides of the spectrum. Remember, science and medicine will always change and evolve. This is especially true when grappling with the less tangible issues such as faith and prayer. So although I have my own thoughts on the subject, I am going to give you both sides of the story. Ultimately, when it comes to faith, it's up to you to decide what's compelling.

Let's begin with two of the most remarkable studies of intercessory prayer. In the first study, 395 patients in a coronary care unit were divided into two groups. Half the patients were prayed for by volunteers. Neither the doctors nor the patients knew who was being prayed for. Patients in the prayed-for group had significantly lower rates of heart failure. None of them required artificial ventilation, compared to 12 patients in the non-prayed-for-group who required it. And they developed fewer complications overall.

Though these results were certainly interesting, the medical world did not really take note until the prestigious *Archives of Internal Medicine* published the results of another study of intercessory prayer and healing. A team of researchers at St. Luke's Hospital in Kansas City, Missouri, led by William Harris, Ph.D., examined the health outcomes of nearly 1,000 newly admitted patients with serious cardiac conditions.

The patients were randomly assigned to one of two groups. Those in one group were prayed for once a day by five volunteers. The volunteers believed in God and in the healing power of prayer, but the patients themselves weren't told they were being prayed for, or even that they were in a scientific study. Patients in the second group didn't receive prayers from the volunteers. The people doing the praying never met the patients. They were told only their first names, and they never visited the hospital. They were only instructed to pray for the patients' "speedy recovery with no complications."

The group receiving the prayers had fewer chest pains and less pneumonia and infection than those who weren't prayed for. They were less likely to die after their treatments. Overall, they did 11 percent better than the non-prayer group. Admittedly, this isn't a huge difference, but it's what scientists call "statistically significant"—the numbers were too high to be attributable merely to chance. Critics of this study point out that the patients in both groups stayed in the hospital for the same lengths of time, meaning that the prayer for a "speedy recovery" didn't pan out. This is a fair criticism, but the study clearly showed *some* difference between the two groups.

As more and more information arose about these scientific studies and intercessory prayer, many in the medical community responded with great skepticism and the methodology of the research was roundly criticized. Although a substantial percentage of the research on prayer has been reported in peer-reviewed scientific journal, there are still many critics of this sort of research. Skeptics rightly note that prayer and faith have a powerful placebo effect. That is, people who pray for health feel better because they *think* prayer works. In virtually every medical study, about a third of participants who are given an inactive substance (a placebo) improve about as much as those given the real treatment. The mind does amazing things, and the placebo effect is a real phenomenon. Yet scientists who study prayer and faith have taken this into account. They've conducted studies in which the placebo effect simply doesn't apply—in studies on laboratory mice, for example, or the growth rate of germs in test tubes. Mice and germs aren't influenced by the power of positive thinking. Yet even in these studies, prayer makes a difference.

In a final attempt to squash the debate on intercessory prayer, a large foundation sponsored a multi-center, rigorously controlled scientific trial called the STEP program. In this study, patients from six of the finest hospitals in the United States were divided into three groups. The first knew that were being prayed for, the second did not know they were receiving intercessory prayer, and the third was a control group (in other words, no one prayed for them). In 2006, the prestigious *American Heart Journal* published the results.

This research showed absolutely no improvement in outcome for either those who received intercessory prayer or those who did not. In fact, those who knew they were being prayed for had a slightly higher complication rate.

As a result of this major study and other smaller studies, most reputable scientists today do not believe that intercessory prayer works in improving health or healing. Perhaps more importantly, most people in the medical community believe that this sort of issue can never be boxed into a purely scientific research project. The control group can never truly be controlled! For those people who were never prayed for, you cannot stop them from praying for themselves or relying on their own faith to serve as their personal support mechanism.

To me, the issue of intercessory prayer is a minor aspect in the relationship between faith and health. You can choose to believe that your prayers will help those in need or that being prayed for will help your own recovery. What's more, you can choose not to believe. From a purely scientific point of view, it may be the process of *believing* that keeps you healthy.

Apart from religious beliefs, quite a few theorists have proposed mechanisms that might explain how prayer works. In a paper published in *Scientific American*, David Chalmers, Ph.D., a cognitive scientist at the University of Arizona, Tucson, suggests that consciousness is a fundamental element of the universe, like matter or energy. This consciousness isn't created by human brains, but is a presence independent of us. A religious person might call this type of independent consciousness or presence "God," like the God that exists in everyone. Following this line of thinking, it starts to make sense that prayer and other "outward" forms of human consciousness could manipulate and be connected to the consciousness in everyone else. To boil this down, it means basically that we are all intrinsically connected. By focusing on the health of another, or attempting to repair someone else's ills, you may actually be able to change his or her condition.

Take a look beyond the philosophical dimensions of prayer and we have a pretty good idea of the physiological effect of praying. Prayer reduces the concentration of hormones in the blood that elevate heart rate and blood pressure. It lowers blood sugar and LDL cholesterol, the form that sticks to artery walls and increases the risk of clots and subsequent strokes or heart attacks. It can also decrease the concentration of hormones that cause anxiety. Recent studies have shown that people who pray regularly have lower levels of cytokines, blood proteins released in response to low-level inflammation, and which are thought to be among the underlying causes of cardiovascular disease.

A study funded by the National Institutes of Health reported that people who prayed at least once daily and attended religious services at least once a week were 40 percent less likely to have hypertension than those who prayed or went to church less often. Since high blood pressure is among the leading causes of heart disease, stroke, and kidney failure, I'd be hard-pressed to find a reason why people *shouldn't* embrace their faith or spirituality more fully.

For those who aren't churchgoers, meditation seems to provide a similar response. A study in the *American Journal of Hypertension* reported that teenagers with a high risk of hypertension who meditated twice daily (for 15 minutes a pop) had significant drops in pressure. Even more interesting, the benefits of meditation persisted for several months after the teenagers quit doing it.

The religious life

Beyond the mechanics of being religious—going to church, regular prayer, and belief in God—there are many other elements of living a religious life that impact your health. From community support to religious doctrine, the directive power of religion can often help individuals maintain a healthier life.

People of faith are much less likely to succumb to addictions of any sort than those without religious or spiritual beliefs. Even when they do fall into addiction, they're more likely to recover. It's not by accident that the spiritual basis of the 12 steps of Alcoholic

Anonymous and similar programs is among the most effective strategies for beating addiction. Research studies have shown that merely attending religious services can reduce the risk of alcoholism by about 30 percent. This is true even in those faiths that don't discourage the consumption of alcohol.

For the most part, the more serious you are about your religion or spiritual beliefs, the healthier you'll be and the longer you'll live. For most of us, making healthy lifestyle changes is an uphill battle. It's a lot easier to make these changes if your faith, or peer-pressure within your congregation, family, or neighbors, gives a little extra nudge. This likely explains why people of conservative religious beliefs are generally healthier than those who lean toward more secular points of view. If your faith discourages drinking and smoking, well, that's a powerful incentive. It also explains why people of faith not only tend to take better care of themselves, but also require fewer doctor visits that people without these beliefs.

Many religions promote a "clean" lifestyle. Perhaps the most solid example of the lifestyle element of religion lies in the Seventh-day Adventist Church.

Researchers have been studying the rather remarkable health and longevity of members of the Seventh-day Adventist Church from as far back as the 1970s. The Adventists are uniquely suited for scientific study for two main reasons. First, the church advocates healthy habits. Alcohol and coffee are discouraged. A vegetarian diet is recommended. Most Adventists consume far more antioxidants and dietary fiber than most Americans—and far less disease-causing fat or processed foods. The second thing that makes the Adventists almost an optimal group for study is that they're a relatively homogenous group. People who are born into the faith tend to stay in the faith, and relatively few "outsiders" enter into the faith later in life. This consistency makes them almost a "living laboratory" for scientists who are trying to measure the impact of particular lifestyle factors on such things as disease rates and mortality. As you'd expect, the Adventists' rates of cancer, heart disease, and other "lifestyle" diseases are significantly lower than in the general population.

I suspect that the health of the Adventists is indirectly but inextricably linked to their faith. The Adventist church discourages the consumption of foods that are proscribed as "unclean" in the book of Leviticus (such as pork), and they also believe that it's their religious duty to take care of the bodies that God gave them. It's not just their faith per se that makes them healthy, but the ways in which their faith guides them to a healthier life.

But, living a "clean" or devout life extends beyond alcohol and pork. Studies have shown that the rate of heart disease is much lower in Catholics than in Protestants or Jews, despite the fact that the dietary and lifestyle habits among these groups aren't markedly different. Dig a little deeper and you can find that specific faiths can place importance on a wide array of issues. Catholics tend to place very high importance on self-responsibility, personal achievement, and ambition, personality traits that have been linked to lower rates of disease. Obviously, these qualities are present in people of all faiths, but when you look at populations rather than individuals, there may be a slight edge among certain groups of believers—and this edge can add up to significant differences.

Beyond religion
The universal elements of faith
Up until now, we've focused primarily on the ways in which religion and the guidelines that many religious groups set forth can impact your life. But what about non-believers? What about people who do not ascribe to any religious teachings?

My close colleague Dr. Sandy Pope has studied extensively the key elements of faith that link to health. While attending religious services, believing in a higher power, and studying the bible are linked to better health, they pale in importance to the impact of being good, giving, loving, and forgiving, none of which are limited to believers. Whether you learned these traits through religion or not, the impact of being a *good person* goes a long way in promoting health.

Being good. It is hard to define goodness. Rather, this characteristic is best judged from within. You know if you're a good person. You may attend church or give money and still be a bad person inside. Being good is about doing the right thing whenever you can.

Being loving. Love is the cornerstone of faith. St. Paul famously said that "in the end there are only three things of importance, love, faith, and hope, and of these, the most importance is love." The more you love, the longer you'll live.

Giving. Charity is a requirement of every faith. Give of yourself, your money, and your time, and you'll be a healthier person. People who volunteer two hours a week live longer and have fewer health problems than those who do not. Indeed, the more you give, the better.

Being forgiving. The most powerful link between faith and health is to learn to say you're sorry. Admit mistakes, don't bear a grudge, and let go of whatever plagues you.

<u>Prayer and the non-believer</u>

Prayer arises from the belief that there is something greater and wiser than ourselves, something that can influence our lives and make them better. Most of us think of prayer as something associated only with religions. Christians, Muslims, and Jews pray. But you don't need a religion to tap in to the healing qualities of prayer. Whether you relate to meditation, communing with nature, or simply taking a moment to reflect, all of these actions ultimately help you achieve the same goal. For me, prayer—both as a term and as a practice—is a simple and universal concept.

There's little reason to think that anyone has to believe in God or anything else to benefit from prayer. Why would you pray if you don't believe in God? Well, for the same reasons that religious people pray: Because you know that the universe is a vast, mysterious, and often-lonely place. We all need to know that there's something out there that can help us through our lives.

The only things required for successful prayer are the emotions that are at the heart of virtually every religion and spiritual movement—things like empathy, love, and compassion. Take a look at the Lord's Prayer. The word *I* is nowhere to be found. It's all about love and compassion for others, being part of something larger than ourselves, and being connected on levels that run deeper than conscious thought.

People who pray feel more relaxed, more sure of themselves, and are better able to face the future. The profound relaxation helps curtail the flood of stress hormones that pour from the adrenal glands during times of stress.

Think back to the very first chapter: *More Peace and Less Stress*. Prayer can be considered another form of seeking peace and reducing stress. There are thousands of studies documenting the effects of prayer and the relaxation response. These studies are uniformly positive. Patients who pray or practice other forms of relaxation have less anxiety before surgery and less pain afterward. Prayer and meditation can lower blood pressure markedly. In fact, patients who pray often and generally take an active role in reducing stress can sometimes reduce their doses of blood pressure-lowering drugs. Some are able to discontinue the drugs entirely. There are few parameters of physical health that *aren't* improved by prayer's relaxation response. There are many ways to achieve the health benefits of prayer and it is certainly not limited to the realm of spirituality. However, if you are faithful, learning to pray in a healthful way can certainly add years to your life.

Prayer in practice

I wasn't a praying man until fairly recently in my life. Even today, now that I've embarked on a new, more spiritual phase of life, I still don't pray in any formal sense. But I do make the effort on most days to set aside a minute or two, at least, to give thanks for the things most important to me, and to express my hopes for a better tomorrow. Quite a few of my patients, when we talk about faith and prayer, will say something like, "I don't know where to begin." Neither did I. If you didn't grow up in a religious family, prayer can seem unnatural and awkward at first. Don't let that put you off. The only real requirement is faith—faith that the world can be a better place, and that you can make yourself a better person who inhabits it.

From my perspective, prayer is not necessarily an expression of religious beliefs (although it certainly can be), but something much broader—accessible to everyone, religious and non-religious alike.

In the last few years, I've started asking all of my patients if religion is important in their lives. If they say it is, then I talk about the strong link between their faith and their current and long-term health. Yet many of my patients say no—they're not religious, they don't pray, and they aren't quite sure what to make of my rather personal questions. To put them at ease, I sometimes explain that I'm not particularly religious myself. I consider myself a secular Jew. I have little interest in organized religion, and rarely attend synagogue. I go mainly on the Jewish New Year and the Day of Atonement. Even then, I don't go to pray or ask God for forgiveness. Rather, I feel it's a good time to step back from my hectic schedule and look a little deeper into my inner self.

During the few hours I spend at the synagogue, I often think a lot about my childhood (so long ago!). I remember attending services with my father every Friday night and Saturday morning. Even though I've left many of the traditions behind, I take great pleasure in these memories, in finding a link that extends back not only to my father, but to the generations that came before. These are the memories that bring me to the synagogue on the high holidays. I always wear my father's prayer shawl (*tallis*) and his skullcap (*yarmulke*). It makes me feel connected—to myself, to my family, and to my cultural roots.

Like most of us, I experienced some profound changes in the wake of the terrorist attacks of September 11. My daughter, a junior at Pomona College in California, was spending the year learning Chinese in Beijing. The attacks devastated her and the other American students with her. They were out of their culture, strangers in a strange land, and living with people who couldn't fully understand their shock and loss. It was then that my daughter, for the first time, turned back to her faith and began meeting with a rabbi.

A year later she had her bat mitzvah, a coming-of-age ceremony that she conducted entirely in Hebrew. I was overcome with emotion, and I felt, for the first time in many decades, how deeply my faith was embedded in who I am. At about that time, my daughter started concluding our visits with a simple and heartfelt, "May God bless you." It sounded awkward to my out-of-practice ears, and I was a little embarrassed about responding in kind. But I did, and liked the way it sounded. Now, I end every visit with my patients with those same, simple words.

I've come to believe that it's not so much religion or prayer that keep us healthy, but the sense of community we share with each other and with the universe as a whole. Giving thanks for our blessings, and living with humility and integrity are the essence of spirituality. I suppose there are some who pray for vengeance, but the prayers deepest in our hearts are for peace, tolerance, and understanding. The capacity to forgive and be forgiven—that seems to be the key to both a long and happy life.

I'm still not a religious man in the usual sense, but since my daughter's epiphany (and mine), I've become much spiritual. I'm more aware of the presence of God in everything we do. I can't say that I pray in any conventional way, but I find myself full of love for the world we live in. Is that a prayer? I think it is. I believe I'm a better man for it. And, of course, a healthier one.

Make prayer suit you

Wherever you find yourself on the path to spirituality, I urge you to continue to seek faith in your life. Faith (not necessarily religion) is what keeps us healthy and sustains us in the face of life's challenges. As we age and enter yet another phase of life, embracing your faith becomes ever more challenging and important. But it's all part of a lifelong path to health, happiness, and peace.

Here are five tips to help you develop your own path to prayer:

Do what suits you. There is no rule on how to pray. Use words if that suits you. You can pray for specific outcomes like: "Help me lower my blood pressure," or "Make tomorrow better." Or you can simply say: "Let thy will be done." For some people, words cannot capture the depth of the moment. So sing if you like! Paint, walk, listen to music—do whatever suits *you*.

Choose your prayer. Every religion and spiritual practices includes entire libraries of traditional and non-traditional prayers. In the end, you can pray for whatever moves you. Here are four main types of prayer:

- Conversational prayer, in which you speak on a personal level with God—sharing your feelings, worries, hopes for the future, and so on.

- Meditative prayer, in which you concentrate your mind on a particular word or phrase or simply remove all thoughts in order to relax and induce a state of meditation.

- Petitionary prayer means asking God or a Higher Power for some "favor" or outcome: better health, a happy family, or even a successful business venture.

- Ritualistic prayer means reciting prayers or texts associated with a particular religion: The Lord's Prayer, for example.

Pray alone—at least some of the time. In the Book of Matthew, Jesus instructs his followers to "enter into a closet and when thou has shut thy door, pray to thy father, which is in secret." Jesus apparently thought that prayers should be a personal matter between a person and God. While there obviously isn't any problem with praying in groups or along with a congregation in church, we all need time for peace and solitude. Allow yourself the space to pray alone. This can help bring you closer to the larger things in life. You'll also be more likely to elicit the physiological responses—such as lower blood pressure, a slower heart rate, and a reduced need for oxygen—that are so beneficial for long-term health.

Be honest and sincere. Nothing is off-limits when you're praying. It's the perfect time to unburden yourself of whatever's in your heart, even (or especially) those things that you're embarrassed about or ashamed of. But prayer *must* be totally open and accepting. You must approach prayer with complete honesty and sincerity.

Leave expectations at the door. Honest and thoughtful prayer should not be encumbered with expectations. It's all too common for people new to prayer to wait anxiously for results or answers—as though God will pick up the telephone! It's never that simple. The "answers" to your prayers may come in many different forms. Most times, the "answers" are within, only accessible when we achieve the wisdom and self-knowledge to see them. If you approach prayer with a specific expectation, you almost certainly limit yourself from seeing the true wonders of our world.

CHAPTER 7
LOVE YOURSELF

My wife, Francie, and I met at the University of Kansas Medical School; she was a medical student and I was her professor. Recently divorced from my first wife, I found myself eager to have a healthy, positive relationship. Ultimately, Francie and I got married and moved to Arkansas. As we settled into our new surroundings, we became more involved in the social scene and attended many parties. At each new party I clung to Francie, daunted by the prospect of chatting with unfamiliar people. What would I say? What would we talk about? Why would they care about a young physician and researcher?

Francie, who is the consummate social butterfly, said to me, "If I wanted to be with you all night, I would not have come to this party! Go meet people, make friends!" She forced me out of my shell and, nearly thirty years later, most people would not believe I was ever so shy! Today, I love making friends and socializing; I jump at the opportunity to dive in to unfamiliar situations. I do not even remotely resemble that introverted, quiet physician who was unable to carry on a conversation.

I was not a "different person" back then—I was, rather, in a different place. At that time, I had just endured a gut-wrenching divorce, narrowly escaping the situation and leaving three young children with their mother. For a long time I felt deeply guilty, knowing that my three children suffered greatly and, ultimately, I felt it was my fault. I was unhappy, carried a huge burden of guilt, and was not comfortable in my own skin.

Fortunately, time healed my wounds and I overcame the bouts of insecurity and guilt. But it was not until well into my forties that I truly developed the tools to become a more confident, secure person. Again, my heart attack served as a serious wake-up call for what kind of person I wanted to be and what kind of life I wanted to lead. My therapy not only helped me control stress, it also gave me the space to understand and dissect my own shortcomings and insecurities. Most importantly, I learned to love myself—both the good and the bad. I committed to work on myself, to be a better person, and to live a happier, more confident, and positive life.

Learning to cultivate confidence and self-love was certainly a healthy process, but I could never have predicted it would actually *lengthen my life expectancy*. In recent years, physicians and researchers in the mainstream medical community have come to realize the healing power of high self-esteem and confidence, qualities that are among the most powerful predictors of longevity. The better you feel about yourself, the longer, happier, and healthier your life will be.

The sixth step in my Longevity plan is love yourself *more*. This is not a simple, fluffy sort of mantra. Don't just pat yourself on the back and say, "Of course I love myself!" Because, in truth, most people do not love themselves enough. At some point in your life I am sure that you struggled with low confidence and poor self-esteem. We all have. Part of living a healthy and passionate life is learning to embrace every element of yourself—to love yourself unconditionally and take the good with the bad, the positive with the negative. You'll find that this simple step will certainly make you a healthier and happier individual.

Why don't we love ourselves? Challenges to self-love ...

We live in an incredibly competitive and judgmental society. We constantly strive to get more, do more, and rise higher than those around us. Our worth is measured by what we "do," not who we are. While I'm a big proponent of doing *more*—not less— you have to do more with a healthy reason and a positive motivation. For many Americans, this culture of striving has become all-encompassing and inescapable. Once you reach one goal, another more challenging goal follows quickly and you never get the chance to be happy and content.

What began as a core component of the American dream—to strive, succeed, and excel beyond expectation—has morphed into an ugly cycle of dissatisfaction. It has seeped into every element of our culture, so even children find themselves unhappy and unsatisfied with their accomplishments. In fact, many Americans are unhappy if there is nothing to strive for. Without a clear mission pushing them forward, they find themselves completely depressed. This is the ultimate problem with lack of self-love. You have to be able to love yourself and be content regardless of life's ups and downs.

For me, this message was most clear when working with one of my favorite patients. He was a very successful businessman who had achieved every possible measure of success in building his business. One day I asked him what made him successful and he said, "Never be satisfied. Never rest on your laurels, because there is always a way to improve and be better." Clearly, this strategy worked well. Had he been content with the success of one store, he may never have seen the growth of the second or third or one-hundredth! His striving approach to life offered everything he could need to be happy and content … until he was forced to retire. Upon retirement, he saw nothing to strive for, nothing to achieve. And, as a result, he was incredibly, irrevocably depressed. During all those decades of success, he only found happiness in the challenge to grow his business. By the time I knew him, at age 85, he had already dwindled into a very poor state of health. It was the price he paid for success.

His story offers a message to all of us, myself included. In the face of retirement and a new chapter in life, many baby boomers will face a huge challenge to be happy without the job or career or success that has defined us. This is where loving yourself *more* comes in. Learn to love yourself and be content regardless of what you do or where you are. If you only define yourself on what you do and what you accomplish, you will never find true contentment.

Why self-love?

The definition of self-love is very similar to self-esteem. However, there are some distinct differences. Both terms refer to a deeply seated emotional understanding that *you can cope with life's challenges* and are *worthy of happiness*. Self-esteem is a very finite and limited definition, while self-love can be variable and multi-faceted. Self-love is more about your ability to be kind to yourself in the face of failure or defeat. You may not identify with having low self-esteem, but everyone can identify with having periods without self-love.

People who love themselves are confident of success, feel loved by those around them, and are contented with their lives (not coincidentally, they usually have a good body image). Conversely, people without self-love often have a negative self-image, find themselves unattractive, lack confidence, and may be described as shy. A poor self-image relates negative thoughts about yourself—always feeling like a failure or unlovable.

The picture of a person without self-love varies greatly. Not always the classic "shrinking violet," people with low self-love are often workaholics and are highly competitive. Underneath a strong exterior, a person with low self-love is often extremely critical of everything. Low self-love often contributes to dysfunctional relationships and destructive behaviors. In extreme cases, people without self-love do not take care of themselves, have few friends and are often alone.

Low self-esteem: a serious health risk
Having low self-esteem is a very serious health issue and some believe that it has all the hallmarks of a life threatening disease. The common symptoms that characterize this condition are uncontrollable, not dissimilar from a patient suffering from depression, anxiety, or heart disease. Low self-esteem is a potent predictor of a shorter life expectancy and a high risk of illness in late life. It is associated with a higher risk of suicide and addictive behaviors such as alcoholism, drug addiction, gambling, compulsive spending, and promiscuity. Low self-esteem may even be the root cause of many forms of criminal behavior, including burglary, violent crimes, sexual assaults, and white-collar crimes.

Why we don't love ourselves ...

Throughout our lives, there are many different issues, encounters, and situations that can impact your own sense of self-love and self-esteem. Each individual has his or her own challenges to address. However, these are three major culprits that typically affect your capacity for self-love—your childhood, feelings of guilt, and unhealthy relationships.

<u>Your childhood</u>
Compelling evidence shows that the source of low self-love may be rooted in your childhood. And it makes sense. Of course you will be forever impacted by your parents!

Tracing a lack of self-love to your childhood can lead to a huge array of issues, from the obviously damaging to the seemingly more benign. Perhaps you were verbally, physically, or sexually abused. Or perhaps you did not feel loved or nurtured at home. Your home environment may have been very rigid and disciplined, where no one expressed their emotions. Perhaps no one ever told you they loved you, or expectations were excessively high. All of these factors can impact and undermine your overall sense of self worth and self-love.

But your childhood situation does not have to be so obviously negative to damage your feelings of self-love and self-esteem. As you know, dysfunctional families come in all shapes and sizes. The most damaging situations are often those that happen behind the perfect picture of smiling faces, parents who present one reality to the outside world and another behind closed doors. This can place a huge pressure on a child to uphold a false picture of perfection. Perhaps your parents were workaholics, leaving you with little support and direction. Or your parents may have been so driven that it left you with a skewed definition of success. Also, children who have experienced their parents divorce often have an impacted sense of trust and relationships, which can in turn contribute to a lack of self confidence later in life.

In addition to the impact your parents can have on your self-worth and self-image, your childhood experiences outside of the home can also affect your feelings of self-love. We all have stories of childhood bullies or the "mean girls" of high school infamy. But for some people the taunting or pressures they felt in school left a long-lasting impact on their own self-image. Again, this can come in many different forms. It is not just the nerdy fat kid that is negatively impacted by the school bully. In high school, I knew a young woman who seemed the image of perfection. She excelled in both academics and sports. She had the classic, enviable high school experience: she was the most popular girl in school, she dated the most handsome boys, and she did it all with a smiling, considerate demeanor. How lucky! To top it off, she came from the classic perfect family. But underneath the shining exterior, she was terribly unhappy. She felt constrained by the pressure to be the perfect high school student. She constantly strove to uphold this image she created and never felt that she was truly "herself." Unknown to anyone at the time, she was bulimic and depressed. She even dealt with self-mutilation. Today, over 50 years later, she continues to struggle with feelings of depression and has spent decades cultivating self-love.

Although her story seems extreme, it provides a lesson for all of us, regardless of age. Sometimes our childhood scars stay with us forever. Learning to love yourself from a young age will offer lifelong benefits.

Guilt

As a Jewish boy, guilt is an emotion with which I am acutely familiar. If Catholic mothers are master inflictors of guilt, my mother has a PhD! Each week I call my mother and simply say, "I'm sorry!" I know I've done *something* wrong. I forgot to call my sister on her birthday. I did not send my mother the medications I promised. I was late calling last week.

My mother makes statements like, "Thank God your father is not alive to see this," or "with a son like you, no wonder I have high blood pressure." But my all-time favorite comment is: "David, you definitely are my brightest child, but you are not my favorite!" How could I ever respond to that?

Before I get too wrapped up in guilt, I have to think about why my mother does what she does. Ultimately, I came to realize she uses this tactic with specific goals in mind:

1. Never ever forget the importance of your family, always love them and be considerate.

2. You can always try to be a better person.

3. Remember that the most important woman in your life is your mother!

In the end, my mother's guilt amuses me. She is never demeaning and always quick to forgive. Her guilt is "good guilt." This is distinctly different from the guilt I felt when divorcing my first wife and leaving three young children. That sort of guilt was "bad guilt," the kind that stayed with me and weighed on my conscience.

The guilt I felt after ending my marriage affected every relationship I had and even impacted my day-to-day work. The guilt that I felt was completely self-imposed; it brought along an inner voice that told me I did not deserve to be happy. It added, "I failed at my first marriage, so why should I succeed in my second?" I even thought, "I'm a bad father and a bad person."

This inner dialogue was devastating. I constantly put myself down and undermined my own path to happiness. It was not until I began to understand the destructive nature of guilt and recognize my own lack of self-love that I could begin to repair relationships and grow.

Many of us have experienced this sort of guilt, whether it was circumstantial or more pervasive, from an inner voice or an outer one. Ultimately, all guilt is self-imposed. Regardless of how and why your guilt developed, you are responsible for the impact it can have on your life. You may or may not have done something wrong, but the truly bad guilt permeates your being and creates a strong inner voice that weighs-in on nearly every decision, thought, or action. The antithesis of self-love, this voice of negativity undermines your own personal barometer for what is good or bad, possible or impossible; it compromises your outlook on life. By dropping the inner dialogue, you can assess each situation as it is and act appropriately. Freeing yourself from guilt is not the same as freeing yourself from responsibility or accountability. If you have done something wrong, apologize and take actions to rectify the situation. But do not let poor decisions or bad choices create a lifelong negativity. Love yourself enough to make mistakes and move on.

<u>Unhealthy relationships.</u>
Relationships of any kind can have an extremely positive or an extremely negative impact on your self-love. Your relationship with your spouse, your friends, your children, and even your co-workers can all affect your attitude toward life. If you already have a propensity for poor self-image, personal relationships are a prime area for unhealthy dynamics. If you do not value yourself or your inherent goodness, you open the door to other people who do not value you as well. This can often result in an emotionally or physically abusive relationship. Alcoholism, gambling, drug addiction, and infidelity can irrevocably harm relationships, which can in turn shake your own foundation of self-love.

Beyond intimate relationships, unhealthy dynamics can exist in any interpersonal relationship. Perhaps you have an abusive co-worker, an insulting supervisor, or a harassing and uncomfortable workplace. Or you may have the pressure of being a caregiver to a dependent spouse, relative, or child. All of these situations have the potential to create stressful dynamics that can affect your own stability.

The health of a relationship hinges on one main thing: *trust*. Like guilt, this one issue always comes back to *you*. If you cannot trust yourself, you certainly cannot trust another. Without self-love and being confident in your own skin, you will never experience the transformative power of trust. Ultimately, this is connected directly with vulnerability. If you cannot trust, you cannot be vulnerable. Without being vulnerable, you cannot truly open yourself to another human being. This is where unhealthy, negative relationships are formed.

The measure of a good relationship is your ability to share your vulnerabilities and your deepest fears, a concept that's the opposite of how many American men are trained to think. The stereotypical American male frequently sees himself in the mold of John Wayne or the Marlboro Man—born leaders who are ready to take charge and give orders; they expect obedience and do not tolerate weakness. These men are tough, cannot admit mistakes, refuse to say sorry, and, of course, never cry.

But this is a recipe for disaster! Rather than laying the foundation for healthy relationships and love, these stereotypical characteristics lead to problems. Without vulnerability, neither partner has the true potential to grow and succeed in the relationship. Without vulnerability and openness, it is nearly impossible to create a healthy relationship.

Learning to love yourself is the first step to forming healthy relationships with everyone around you. By loving yourself, you will have enough self-worth to eliminate any unhealthy characters in your life. What's more, you will have the insight to choose a friend or a partner who is safe, solid, and trustworthy. With sufficient self-love, you will not be dependent on another human being to make you happy. You can be happy on your own! By committing to this philosophy, you not only allow yourself to be happy, but you also allow your friends and loved ones to be themselves, unencumbered by expectations or the pressures of an unhealthy relationship.

Do you lack self-love?

A good way to determine if you have a poor self-image or lack self-love is to complete a questionnaire either online or in a book. Here is an abridged screening test that may be helpful. It is a shortened version of a self-compassion scale developed by Kristin Neff, Ph.D., at the University of Texas at Austin.

Most of the time…

1. When I'm feeling down, I tend to feel like most other people are probably happier than I am.

2. When I think about my inadequacies, it tends to make me feel more separate and cut off from the rest of the world.

3. When I'm feeling down I tend to obsess and fixate on everything that's wrong.

4. When I'm really struggling, I tend to feel like other people must be having an easier time of it.

5. I'm intolerant and impatient towards those aspects of my personality I don't like.

6. When something painful happens I tend to blow the incident out of proportion.

7. When I fail at something that's important to me, I tend to feel alone in my failure.

If you answered yes to five of these questions you likely lack self-love and should consider seeking help.

Ten steps to loving yourself *more*.
Here are my 10 simple steps to empower yourself to improve your feelings of self worth, confidence and self-love.

1. Work hard on improving your self-image.

Americans have an unhealthy obsession with our physical appearance. We are so envious of those beautiful and buff bodies that cover the pages of every magazine, monopolize our television sets, and are promoted as the "most beautiful people in the world." Why are film stars and celebrities, with their propensity to excess, addiction, promiscuity, and multiple marriages, our role models? Everyone I know—regardless of age or waistline—seeks to "get into shape." Whose shape are we trying to get into? What has happened to our country? We must all see the beauty in ourselves and in others. By loving yourself more, you can free yourself from this pressure to fit into someone else's idea of the perfect man or woman. By loving yourself more, you will emanate beauty from every pore.

Here are some approaches to consider:

- Every day, stand naked in front of a full-length mirror and tell yourself that you're gorgeous. At first it may be hard to do, but with time it will become easier. Don't look at those extra pounds and think negative thoughts. Remember there is nothing wrong with being pleasantly plump.

- Look closely at your face in the mirror. Look for those wrinkles, crows' feet, blemishes on your face, and bags under your eyes, and tell yourself you have grace and beauty, you are wise and measured and a true sage.

- Never pass a mirror without looking at yourself and saying "aren't I cute!"

- Always see the beauty in those around you. Tell your partner how beautiful he or she is and how good they look.

- Do whatever makes you feel beautiful. Seek advice from a fashion expert and buy clothes that fit and make you look and feel attractive. Do things that make you feel better about yourself, whether it is exercising, volunteering, joining a gym, or taking an art class.

2. Make sure your needs are met.

It's amazing how we disregard ourselves and our needs. Even when surrounded by others, we are often alone. Know yourself well enough to recognize your own needs and desires. Everyone is different and we all have specific actions or tools to help us soothe and center during difficult times. Know what those are and make time to do them!

Here are some suggestions:

- Make time to eat right and exercise every day. Make sure that you don't eat on the run. Sit down and have a meal with your family.

- Learn to say no. Don't take on too many tasks that are over-whelming. Only do things you really want to do, and avoid approaching any task feeling that this is something you have to—rather than want to—do.

- Don't burn the candle at both ends. Working or playing too hard leads to stress, exhaustion, and an increased risk of failure.

- Make time for things that are fun and that you enjoy. Don't be so busy that you never have any fun. Go out to dinner with friends, go to a movie or an art show, take a stroll! Make a list of things you really enjoy and go do them.

- Take vacations. Studies show that vacations are highly beneficial to your health. So, go away. Remove yourself from the stressors of daily life and take some time to get balanced.

3. Work on seeing the good in you and those around you.

Lack of self-love always presents itself in a negative outlook and at-titude about yourself or those around you. It is extremely vital that you develop a healthy, positive inner voice. By focusing on the good in you and in those around you, any situation can be improved and you are more likely to find a positive resolution to problems.

Here are some approaches to consider:

- Identify all of your positive attributes. This may be the way you look, the color of your eyes, your smile or your quick mind, intellectual or physical skills, or activities in which you excel. Then identify those attributes you view as negative. Combine the list and you should see a very balanced person, with both good and bad qualities. Work on loving the total package.

- Work on being comfortable with yourself. Set your own measures of success.

- Become realistic about yourself and stop driving yourself to be perfect. Set attainable and reasonable goals for yourself.

4. Learn to reward yourself for a job well done.
A cardinal feature of poor self-love is dissatisfaction with your accomplishments. Nothing is ever good enough and "it can always be better." This inability to find contentment is a direct reflection of your own insecurities. By learning to love yourself more, you can find peace in the little things as well as the big. Here are some suggestions.

- Do the best you can and let that be enough. Try to see that others are doing the best they can as well.

- Work hard to finish a task that you initiate. Take criticism constructively and not personally. Often it is meant to help rather than harm.

- Celebrate your accomplishments! Feel happy about what you have done; treat yourself to something special. Don't wait for some huge event to celebrate; find happiness in the little things and let others find happiness in them as well.

- Be contented with where you are right now. Stop looking to the future or to past with longing or anticipation.

This only takes you away from the present. Work on being happy with this simple moment. Treat each day as if it were your last.

5. Eradicate negativity.

Lack of self-love is almost always accompanied by negativity about everything—individuals, your job, your accomplishment, the movies, restaurants. Even your thought processes become negative. Therefore, eradicating negativity is an enormous step in this process. Consider the following:

- Eliminate the negative words in your life! Words carry great weight, so if you can approach situations with a positive phrase or positive speech it will certainly impact everyone around you. Be careful with your words and try to remain as positive as possible.

- If the answer is "I can't," ask yourself why. Sometimes it is okay to say no, but if the reason is lack of confidence, give it a whirl and say, "I can."

- Listen to yourself and stop the negative thoughts. You are not a bad person, you are not stupid, you are not a klutz, and you are worthy of love.

- Take a break to consider your thoughts. Are you unduly critical? Would you say the same thing of someone else? Most likely, the answer is no and you will find that you are unnecessarily tough.

- If you have a negative thought about yourself, ask someone you trust and see if they feel the same way. This may help you view yourself differently. The key to this step is being open to the possibility that you may be wrong.

6. Stop judging.

Those without self-love are constantly judging everyone around them. Denigrating others is often a way to overcome your own feeling of inadequacy. It is imperative to start catching those judgments each time they pop up. By first noticing when and how you judge, and then actively dissecting that thought, you will slowly begin to be less judgmental. Consider these tips:

- Avoid discussing your negative impressions about others with anyone.

- Be very measured and careful about criticism. Dwell on your thoughts for a while before making your opinions known. If you criticize, be constructive.

- If you are unhappy with someone, discuss it with them directly. Although confrontation is uncomfortable, dealing with conflicts the right way makes for a better resolution.

- Avoid water-cooler gossip. Don't be devious, don't exaggerate, tell the truth, and avoid pitting one person against another either in the home or work setting.

7. Work on building trust.

Many of us are suspicious of those around us, particularly if we have been seriously hurt. Whether it be the unfaithful husband, an insensitive child, or a colleague at work, developing trust and understanding with others is essential. Remember, the single most powerful characteristic of a good individual is your capacity to forgive. Consider these suggestions:

- Begin with yourself. Be vulnerable and honestly understand how and why you feel a certain way. If you can develop a trusting relationship with yourself, only then can you develop a trusting relationship with others.

- Trust others. Jealousy is like a cancer that destroys trust and relationships. Trust those around you to do the right thing. If you can't, the relationship will surely fail.

- Don't bury conflicts under the rug. Discuss them and try to resolve them, either together or with help. Conflict resolution may require a mediator or a therapist.

- Forgive, forgive, forgive. You can never move forward without truly forgiving the other party and yourself.

- Let go. Allow yourself and those around you to have as much freedom as possible.

8. Avoid bad relationships.

Many individuals with low self-love have been surrounded by bad relationships all their lives. Without self-love, it's easy to end up in dysfunctional marriages, become codependent, or drift to friends who have emotional problems. This feeds a very unhealthy cycle that leads to unhappiness and ever worsening self-esteem. So how do you know that you are in a bad relationship? Begin with following questions.

- Are you getting what you need from the relationship?

- Are you being taking advantage of or are ignored?

- Do you feel you never communicate?

- Do you perpetually feel unsatisfied?

- Do you feel continuously stressed and anxious when your mate is around?

- Is your relationship filled with lies, lies and more lies?

- Is your partner controlling or emotionally and physically abusive?

- Is your partner never home?

If the answer to some or all of these questions is *yes*, you may have a significant problem. The problems may be very obvious or very subtle, but either situation creates a negative impact on your personal health. If you find yourself in unhealthy relationships, seek help. Make sure that you are not making excuses for yourself or your partner. Always do what's best for you and do not be afraid to ask your partner to grow. Be honest. People are resilient and have an amazing ability to adapt. By being honest and vulnerable, you will certainly find the core of your relationship. However, if you make sacrifices, excuses, or tolerate problems, everyone will suffer.

9. Understand the destructive nature of bad habits.
We all have bad habits. But, when a person lacks of self-love, bad habits often become very destructive tools to undermine personal self-worth. Drug addiction and other compulsive behaviors such as gambling, shopping, overeating, and promiscuity are all negative consequences of poor self-love. If you have negative habits that undermine your own happiness, you must take every step to understand your problem and find a solution.

10. Get involved.
In a world where we are so independent and hurried, sometimes we need to stop and remember that we are all connected. An important element of improving your own self-love is to get involved. Give of yourself to others and you will likely find a deeper, healing connection to humanity.

- Become a volunteer. There is good evidence that individuals who volunteer live longer and are happier than those who do not. It is an important way to meet people and provide a needed service.

- Make an effort to make friends. Join a group and get involved in activities where you have the chance to meet and socialize with people who have interests similar to yours.

- If religion is important in your life, stay active in your spiritual community, participate in services, volunteer and make an effort to attend social gatherings.

- Remain a lifelong learner. Go back to college, attend classes, get involved in any activity that can help you grow, stay involved and connected.

- Become a mentor for a young person and help them learn and grow.

Seek help

If you have struggled with a lack of self-love for a prolonged period of time, overcoming these deeply imbedded impressions of yourself takes much time and effort. Seeking help from a qualified therapist can offer huge benefits. If you have problems with relationships, difficulty in your work setting, or are generally unhappy and negative about yourself, therapy can prove life-saving.

Learning to truly love yourself is a challenging task and often a long journey. Many of us have spent years developing defense mechanisms and negative habits that all contribute to poor self-worth. Of course it will take time to unravel those issues and adopt a healthier approach to life and love. Learning to love yourself will have ramifications that spread across every element of your life.

CHAPTER 8
MORE OF THE RIGHT FOODS

I come from a food-loving people. Growing up in South Africa, my mother cooked traditional Jewish fare, from pickled herring and smoked salmon to gefilte fish and my personal favorite, *tsimis*, a stew containing brisket, vegetables, tons of prunes, and a unique sweet sauce. Our family celebrated around food and enjoyed each other over meals. Today some of my greatest memories involve eating.

Admittedly, my relationship with food has not always been positive. At times, perhaps, I enjoyed food a little too much and my weight reached unhealthy levels. Other times, I looked to food for comfort; eating was a means to an unhealthy end, not a process to be enjoyed and valued. I, too, have been sucked in by the pressures of our image obsessed culture and fallen prey to the diet industry.

I dieted, it failed; I dieted again, and it failed again! Believe me, I know what it is like to be overweight, unhappy, and to fear food. It took me years to realize that food is not the enemy and that diets don't work.

Unfortunately, this is a lesson many Americans have yet to learn. At any given time, 22 percent of American men and 32 percent of American women are on a diet. And yet, nearly two thirds of American adults are overweight—and the problem continues to grow. So, what's wrong?

Here's the secret: the problem with our ever-expanding waistline is more than just about food. It's definitely more than just dieting.

As a nation, we are obsessed with weight loss. Not a day goes by that I don't hear a new story chastising Americans for their growing girth. The American media has launched a very public war on fat. As a result, it has flooded the television, radio, and newspapers with the truth about fat: how fat people are unhealthy, draining the health system, and affecting everyone's bottom line. Scare

Americans into making healthier choices! Right? Wrong. Though their intentions may be good, their solution is not.

Rather than helping Americans understand *health*, this only helps us fear fat. We completely ignore the real truth that fat is not the culprit! Obesity is a result of many things, diet being only one among them. Rather than addressing the cultural, emotional, and societal reasons behind our growing girth, we focus solely on food. This just further encourages an unhealthy relationship with food.

So forget the war on fat. Don't rely on everything the media says and accept the responsibility to be educated about nutrition. **The real problem with Americans' growing girth is not just *what* they eat, but *how* they eat.** Every weight-loss book out there can give you a prescription to lose a few pounds, but the challenge lies in developing a healthier relationship with food. This is how you can truly impact your life, your health, and your risk for developing disease.

So it's time to abandon the notion that losing pounds is the key to lifelong health. Eliminate the idea of diets completely. Diets are only about deprivation—and that never works. It is time to stop depriving yourself of good food!

The seventh step of Dr. David's Longevity plan is *more* food! Be passionate about eating and rely on this key principle: more food, not less. More of the "right" foods that fuel your body, burn fat, and boost energy. As soon as you free yourself from the crazy obsession with fat and weight, you'll be well on your way to finding passion in food.

There a three steps to being passionate about food:
1. Free yourself from diets
2. Cultivate a healthy relationship with food
3. Re-center your plate

Free yourself from diets
For Americans, the urge to lose weight does not diminish with age; it is almost as common among 70-year-olds as it is among

20-year-olds. Even my grandmother used to say, "You can never be too thin or too rich!" And, my daughter thinks she can always lose five pounds. No matter what I say, she refuses to hear me! Those of us who are thin want to be thinner, and those who aren't pray for a miracle diet pill. We study weight-loss articles, sign up at expensive health clubs, and worry about *every little* morsel that passes our lips. We pour billions of dollars into the weight-loss industry … and we've made tycoons of the marketing wizards who take advantage of a vulnerable, insecure, overweight population. They sell us diets that don't work, pills that have little or no effect, and various other weight-loss schemes that usually do more harm than good. Dieting and the urge to be skinnier have become so pervasive that even young children are succumbing to the pressure.

And yet we keep gaining weight. So what is there to do?

My answer is simple: *stop stressing*! Free yourself from diets and don't focus on your weight! Commit to living a healthy lifestyle and your body will find its own ideal weight. At the end of the day, you may still be five to ten pounds over your "prescribed" weight, but who cares? It does not matter! Being slightly overweight is the least important predictor of health and longevity. There are scientific reasons (in addition to emotional reasons) for not agonizing over every extra pound.

A word about obesity

As an empowered consumer of healthcare, it is vital that you distinguish between moderately overweight and morbidly obese. Research done by Dr. Richard Troiano, now with the Centers for Disease Control and Prevention, has found that only *morbid obesity*, and not moderate amounts of extra weight, significantly shortens life expectancy. A close analysis of decades of medical research suggests that there's only a modest connection between health problems and moderate weight gain that tends to occur as we age.

In the end, I encourage any tactic that helps Americans adopt a healthier lifestyle. Just don't buy in to the hype that fat and unhealthy are synonymous.

The war on fat

The focus on the "obesity epidemic" really began with a series of studies. In 1999, the first study published in the *New England Journal of Medicine* examined the role of obesity in increased risk of illness and death. Following 115,000 women who participated in the Women's Health Study, researchers from Harvard Medical School used sophisticated statistics to demonstrate "even mild to moderate overweight is associated with a substantial increase in premature death."

Unfortunately, these researchers greatly overstated their results. Their sophisticated statistics only showed that weight affected life expectancy if they excluded the more overwhelmingly important impact of lifestyle habits, including cigarette smoking, lack of exercise, high blood pressure, elevated cholesterol, and the role of dietary and other factors that can lead to cancer and heart disease. This study also failed to incorporate variances in diet. Both high-fat and high-carbohydrate diets are likely to have an increased risk of heart disease and stroke, but the effect is the same on skinny and fat people alike.

Those who believe obesity is the cause of all our health woes continue to warn that being overweight was the number-one health threat facing our nation. Yet still there is controversy. In a consensus conference sponsored by the National Institutes on Health, a significant number of research scientists led by Dr. Elizabeth Barret maintained that weight was not a significant risk factor for an elevated cholesterol and heart disease. In 2005, the Centers for Disease Control downgraded the number of American deaths directly caused by obesity to 112,000—a very small number. The moral of the story is that your health is more than your weight and being healthy is not limited to a specific pant size.

Why diets fail

The success rate of most diets is less than five percent. Think about that. Out of 100 people who try to lose weight, only five will be successful.

Why is it so hard to lose weight? Ultimately, the answer includes both physiological and psychological reasons.

From your body's perspective, dieting is hard. When your intake of calories drops, the body's metabolism changes to adjust to reduced food consumption. In other words, your body doesn't need as many calories as it did before. This makes sense in evolutionary terms, because the slowdown in metabolism helped keep people alive during lean times. However, it drives modern dieters crazy because losing weight is agonizingly slow.

In addition, when you diet, your body experiences a rapid loss of glycogen, a calorie-rich sugar stored in muscle. As glycogen levels fall, so does the muscles' water concentration. The water loss can be substantial, contributing to 10 pounds or more of weight loss in a single week. This explains why diets that severely restrict calories can produce quick and dramatic weight loss. But here's the rub: glycogen is just as easily replaced as depleted. As soon as you start eating reasonable amounts of food, glycogen and water flood back into the muscles. This is the problem with most diets. When you lose weight rapidly, you are not losing fat. You're losing water. Water is easily replaced and the weight comes right back. Remember, anything that is easy to take off is twice as easy to put on!

Except for those rare individuals with almost superhuman dedication, nearly everyone starts and stops diets. In either case, the pounds rapidly return and you end up disheartened and dejected. This cycle of on-again, off-again dieting is terribly hard on the body … not to mention the mind!

While there are physiological factors that impact your weight-loss plans, the greatest problem with dieting involves emotional and social elements. First, consider the mere fact that at any given time one-fifth the American population is on a diet. Dieting has become a culture unto itself, something everyone "does" without the real commitment to lifestyle change. There are people who are perpetually "on a diet." Now there are even social pressures to be on a diet!

A friend's book club is a terrific example. Ten women all congregate together for lunch and discussion. And yet no one eats! At the beginning of the lunch, one woman clearly states she's "on a diet" and "just couldn't splurge." Of course, the other women follow suit! The thought is: "If *she's* on a diet and she's skinnier than me, then I definitely should be on a diet!" They just look at the food and nibble on whatever seems healthiest. While this alone is ridiculous, the best part of the story is after the book club ends, when half of the women sneak off to their cars for a cigarette and the other half rush home to curb their feelings of starvation and splurge in solitude!

For many men and women today, dieting is the norm. Every day is a day "on a diet." Ultimately, this has many negative effects. First, the diet is always food-focused (if not in name only). Cut calories, deprive yourself, and weight comes off. However, the necessary lifestyle changes are never truly implemented, so the "diet" inevitably fails. Then, because the diet failed and you clearly did not stay in that size-six dress, you feel ashamed and guilty. This just furthers feelings of a negative self-image, prompting many of us to diet again, to fail again, and launching a highly destructive cycle.

In addition to the negative culture of dieting, many people diet for unhealthy reasons. The motivation behind the diet is short term or superficial. Maybe you really want to fit into a new pair of pants or your college reunion is coming up so you want to look your best. Maybe your daughter told you to diet because "you look fat" or maybe it's a new year and you resolved to get back into "pre-parenthood" weight. Honestly, these motivations might get you started, but they aren't good enough to keep you going. More often than not, because the goals are short-term, the diet is short-term as well. You search for the quick-fix diet, not the slow, arduous path to lifelong weight maintenance. Even if you do lose some weight, the odds are you will gain it back—quickly.

Anytime the motivation to lose weight is superficial or vain, your diet is doomed to fail. Truthfully, most Americans fall into this category! The motivation to lose weight is about looking like the models on magazines, impressing someone else, or striving to reach some ridiculous standard that you put on yourself. This is the root of why diets fail. It's not just about the food, or even the exercise: it's about how you feel about yourself. Food must be part of an overall, comprehensive healthy lifestyle. By becoming too obsessed with dieting, many Americans have lost sight of what it means to be healthy.

The upside on plus-size
There are some upsides to being plus-size! This is especially true as you grow older. From the early 1970s, Dr. Reuben Andres, director of the National Institute on Aging's clinical branch, examined the effect of longevity of the population at large. He clearly showed that people who are 10 to 15% overweight tend to have *lower* mortality rates. People who were significantly underweight (10-15% below their ideal body weight) and those who were morbidly obese had a significantly shorter life expectancy. It is possible that those who are on the extremes of the spectrum (either drastically below or above their ideal weight) are more likely to have unhealthy lifestyle habits such as smoking, lack of exercise, or poor nutrition.

Even more recently, a study published in 2005 by Dr. Katherine Flegal from the Centers for Disease Control showed that those who are chubbier live longer. In this report, weight and longevity are inversely correlated. In other words, the heavier you are, the longer you're likely to live. . No one really knows why, but for the population at large being pleasantly plump promotes longevity. A little extra fat may actually confer a survival advantage! This U-shaped curve of longevity clearly shows that either end of the spectrum is more likely to have shorter life expectancy, whether you're significantly overweight or significantly underweight. A little chubby in the middle and your life expectancy is longer!

In 2007 Dr. Flegal and her colleagues published a second paper in the *Journal of the American Medical Association* in which they reiterated their earlier observation that overweight individuals had a longer life expectancy than those who were either very obese or significantly underweight. In this second study, they confirmed the earlier findings and expanded them to examine the causes of death in the three groups. And finally in 2009 an analysis of over 13,5000 Canadians found that those who were overweight but not morbidly obese or very thin lived longer even than those individuals who were at their ideal body weight

Researchers found that being overweight (not obese) was associated only with excess mortality from diabetes and kidney disease. More surprisingly, being overweight was not associated with increased deaths from heart disease or cancer. There was an apparent protective effect for overweight and obese individuals against many other illnesses, including Alzheimer's, various neurological diseases, many infections, chronic lung disease, and injury. The group who were obese had an increased risk of dying from cancers that have been proven to be obesity related, including colon, breast, prostate and kidney cancer.

In addition, a number of studies suggest that people who are somewhat overweight are less likely to develop osteoporosis. After age 75, bone loss is a major cause of dependency among the elderly, contributing to more than 1.5 million hip fractures annually. It has been estimated that more women die of osteoporosis-related conditions than from cancer of the breast, cervix, and uterus combined. Men and women who are slightly overweight exert more daily stress on their bones and as a result their bones are stronger. This is doubly true if regular exercise is included.

Studies also suggest that being overweight may reduce the risk of certain cancers, particularly lung cancer. Researchers have traditionally thought that this protective effect might be an illusion, because people who smoke tend to be thin. But both smokers and nonsmokers have a lower risk of cancer when they are chubbier. In the end, it is a mystery. But for the chubby among us, who cares why it works?

Again, the bottom line is that weight is not a major predictor of risk of death or dying. The "obesity epidemic" has been somewhat overstated, but only insofar as it places too much emphasis on pounds and waistlines. It is possible to be healthy and overweight, fit and fat. Your lifestyle is much more important than your pants size.

Believe me, it's a hard line to sell! But it's true

In a landmark study published in the Journal of the American Medical Association (JAMA) in 2005, Dr. Katherine M. Flegal showed that being underweight was a far greater risk factor for a shorter life expectancy than either being overweight or moderately obese. This information was also obtained from NHANES data and has been summarized in a number of reports issued by the CDC.

The risk of death in individuals of varying health status based on their weight.

	Underweight		Overweight		Moderately Obese	
Age (years)	25-69	70+	25-69	70+	25-69	70+
Excellent or very good health	1.33	1.74	0.91	0.90	1.01	1.02
Good, fair or poor health	1.74	1.65	0.85	0.91	1.05	1.00

In this table the risk of dying is expressed as an odds ratio. A value of 1 means that risk of dying is not increased. A value greater than one means the risk is increased. A value lower than one means the risk is reduced. For example a value of 2 means that you have a 200% increased risk of dying. And if the value is 0.9 your risk of dying is reduced by 10%

The truth about weight and health

The medical and scientific community has spent decades trying to understand the relationship between weight and health. The results have been varied and not everyone agrees on exactly how each extra pound affects your overall health. In the end, the wide array of information is enough to make you stop and think about our fixation on fat. Here are two scientific examples of why it's time to end the obsession with weight loss:

- First, two large studies have documented the effects of weight on long term health. Both the long-running Framingham study and a population survey called NHANES II (National Health and Nutrition Examination Survey II, 1976–1980) found the same U-shaped survival curve that Dr. Reuben Andres initially described.

- Second, research has shown that even the link between coronary artery disease and weight is somewhat dubious. Researchers have found, for example, that the severity of coronary artery disease observed during autopsies cannot be linked to body weight. In studies among the living, researchers have examined the insides of the arteries with angiography and failed to find a relationship between the severity of coronary deposits, or atherosclerosis, and weight. One study, in fact, found an inverse relationship between coronary artery disease and body weight. Subjects with the higher body mass indexes tended to have less arterial narrowing. While some studies have found a link between obesity and coronary artery disease, many have not. Large epidemiological studies performed in the United States and Europe fail to prove a connection between weight and heart disease even after following large groups of people for more than 20 years!

Despite this evidence, doctors continue to point to weight as the major problem in American today. But I disagree! The issue with weight and health really relates to your lifestyle. Overweight individuals tend to be more sedentary and eat unhealthy foods. But skinny people have bad habits, too. These confounding factors are far more important than the number of extra pounds. It's time to stop blaming weight and start focusing on disease. **Ask yourself this question: "Do I have a weight problem—or a health problem?"** If you have been to the doctor and ruled out major health concerns such as high cholesterol, hypertension, diabetes, sleep apnea, joint disease, or any other problem that may be affected by weight, you do not have a health problem. Guess what? You don't have a weight problem either! If you haven't figured it out, it is a trick question. **There is no such thing as a weight problem without a health problem.**

I hope the message is clear: free yourself from the shackles of dieting and learn to love food again. This is the way to a healthier relationship with food, your body, and your health.

Develop a healthy relationship with food

Have you ever heard the saying, "You should eat to live, not live to eat"? While I understand the idea, I must disagree with his philosophy. To "eat to live" implies a very strict relationship with food, where it is no more than fuel for your body and a necessary component of survival. Where is the fun in that? Good food is so much more than fuel: it is an expression of love, culture, and tradition. Developing a passionate and respectful relationship with food is a key component of living a healthy and joyful life.

Finding passion in food relies on the way in which you approach eating: do you eat with a motive? Do you eat because you're sad? Or because you're happy? Do you eat just because food is available? Or because you're bored? For many Americans, food has far surpassed the traditional role of "fuel for the body." More than a necessary element of human survival, the process of eating can accompany a variety of motives, from celebration to commiseration. We all need to recognize that food is not just a necessary part of human survival—it is a privilege to enjoy. The key is developing a healthy relationship with what you eat.

In order to do this, you must first recognize when food provides a means to an unhealthy end.

There are three classic ways in which we develop unhealthy relationships with food. First, viewing **food as fuel**, a necessary part of living, about which we pay little attention. With this sort of concept, we barely even acknowledge the process of eating. We eat on the run, in the car, at our desk, or in front of the television. Food loses all respect. Rather than being an enjoyable, passionate experience, food and eating are secondary to whatever else is going on. This creates an unhealthy relationship because you never really focus on the food you put in your mouth. The satiety that comes with sitting down to enjoy a meal is lost, so you never feel truly satisfied.

The second major culprit that undermines a passion for eating is using **food for comfort**. I can truly identify with this problem. Using food for comfort can come in many forms, from calming nerves to abating boredom, assuaging guilt to soothing loneliness. In my case, I eat when I'm bored. The process of consuming—a handful of cereal, a cup of coffee, or an entire steak—is comforting. I'm not really hungry, but the idea of eating sounds nice. So I eat. I never really feel full or satisfied; in fact, I barely remember eating. Hours later, when sitting down for a meal, you would never know that I had already consumed a scoop of ice cream or a slice of turkey. This is bad … and I know it. But I work on it every day and some days are better than others. But who can't relate to opening the fridge just to see what's available? My unhealthy vice with food is only one example of we use food for comfort. Have you ever heard someone say, "Food is my friend, my confidant"? For some people, food curbs loneliness. It is a trusted friend to turn to when no one else is around. Food can be a source of comfort when you're sad or grieving. I met a patient whose Louisiana home was demolished by Hurricane Katrina. For twelve months she grieved and food was her therapy. Within a year, she had gained sixty pounds and developed a host of health complications.

For anyone who looks to food for comfort, the end result is never quite satisfying. Comfort food never lives up to your expectations and that pint of ice cream typically doesn't make you feel much better. In many cases, you feel worse than when you started, which leads to a very destructive cycle of negativity. By using food as an escape, you fail to acknowledge the real problems.

The final path to an unhealthy relationship with eating is to view **food as the enemy.** People who view food as the enemy fear every calorie, fat gram, or hormone that passes the lips. Fearing food is a very serious issue for millions of Americans and a direct result of our image-obsessed, diet-ridden culture. On the extreme side, fearing food can lead to life threatening eating disorders such as anorexia and bulimia. Men and women afflicted with these disorders see food as the enemy, the cause behind their unhappiness. But people who view food as the enemy are not just those with eating disorders. People simply seeking to lose a few extra pounds can fall prey to this unhealthy mentality. Even some athletes view food as the enemy.

Ultimately, I fear that most Americans fall into this category, especially while the country galvanizes around the "obesity epidemic" but fails to explain fully the entire process of living a healthy life. The end result is a nation full of people afraid to eat! They don't know what is the "right" food instead of the "wrong" food, so anything that is labeled unhealthy gets immediately tossed into the danger pile. Good fat is not distinguished from bad fat; good carbohydrates are not separated from the bad. So by failing to understand what it means to "eat right" or "eat healthy," most Americans face two distinct options: 1) fear most food and adopt a very restrictive diet or 2) give up because fearing food is not sustainable.

I would be shocked to find an American who did not relate to any of these unhealthy approaches to food. If you do not face this challenge personally, I am positive you know someone who does. Regardless of approach, the end result is always the same. Without developing a healthy relationship with food, you can never truly lead a healthy, happy life.

In order to cultivate your own passion for food, begin with these basic steps:
1. Change *how* you eat
2. Educate yourself about food
3. Find your body's natural weight and be okay with it

Change *how* you eat
In order to cultivate a healthy relationship with food, you must change how you eat. This must happen well before you ever start the process of changing *what* you eat. First, **recognize your**

motives for eating. Are you even hungry? How do you hope to feel after your meal? Ultimately, this is about taking stock of your emotions and mindset when it's time to eat. If you have the tendency to eat for comfort or out of boredom, it's vitally important that you recognize that urge and address it. So much of our problem with food is an emotional and mental problem. So learn to notice your motivations. Simply observe your urge to eat. Just by beginning this process of observance, you will naturally start to curb those unhealthy tendencies.

But keep this in mind—developing a healthy relationship with food often means changing lifelong habits. Sometimes you will slip back into those unhealthy tendencies. It's okay. Recognize that you are fallible and make mistakes. If you fall off the bandwagon, do not launch into a guilt-ridden inner dialogue. Simply move forward and try to be better. That is all you can ask.

Second, **slow down**. A key element of developing a healthy relationship with food is actually noticing that you ate! Stop rushing through meals. Stop eating "on the run." Give your food and your body some respect and pay attention to the process of eating. Much of our unhealthy relationship with food comes from our fast-paced, quick-fix culture. But nothing about your health is quick fix. If you are at work, give yourself time for lunch. Take fifteen minutes to step away from your desk, turn off the computer, and eat. This exercise is not only for your emotional health, but your physical health as well. By taking the time to pay attention to eating, you allow your body a chance to regulate and digest in a natural manner. If you eat while performing other tasks especially stressful tasks, you never really allow your body to recognize the process of eating.

Enjoy every bite of food that passes your lips. Pay attention to it! Chew slowly and notice how it tastes and feels. Take a few minutes to eat without talking. Notice everything you can about the process, including how your food looks and smells. How it feels when you're chewing and how your belly feels when you swallow. You may be surprised at what you notice. *The bottom line: give food the respect it deserves!* Don't treat any meal like just a necessary part of survival. Take time to enjoy it. Not only does this have an impact on how you feel about food, it also allows your body to metabolize your meal at a natural pace. Remember, it takes fifteen minutes for your stomach to tell your brain that it's full. By slowing down, you actually consume less food and feel more satisfied. In the end, you have had an enjoyable experience, your belly feels full, and you have likely consumed fewer calories.

The third step in changing how you eat is to **regulate your portion size**. In the last twenty years, portion sizes for the average American meal have grown exponentially. Ultimately, this happened at our request. As consumers, we want more and more for our dollar. Just think about it: if you go to a restaurant and your food is not overflowing on the plate, you feel ripped off! Believe me, if the food industry thought it could serve you less and charge the same, it would. According to statistics from the Centers for Disease Control and Prevention, since 1985 the average number of calories consumed has risen from 1,996 to 2,247 a day. That extra 251 calories a day can work out to an additional 26 pounds per year.

Clearly, portion size is important. But regulating your portions is not about depriving yourself of food, it is about giving your body the amount of food it needs to feel satisfied. It is about eating enough so that you feel neither hungry nor stuffed. Be aware of the fact that restaurants are going to give you too much food. Here are some tips to regulate your portions when eating out:

- Try to eat the amount of food you would eat at home.

- Ask for a to-go box as soon as your food arrives and put half of it away immediately. If you can't see it, you won't eat it. I promise you will not be hungry.

- Ask for a half-portion or split your meal.

- Avoid appetizers and desserts. If you want them, split them with a friend.

- Avoid the bread basket. You don't need all that bread and you will still be compelled to eat all of your meal.

Again, the issue of portion size is not about what you eat, but how you eat. It is more of a mental game than a physical one.

The final step to changing how you eat is **to know your body**. This sounds simple and obvious, but many of us don't listen to our bodies when we eat. Often we eat because our minds tell us to eat, not because our body needs food. So take time to pay attention to your body. Maintain a regular eating schedule, but be kind to your body and don't overdo it. If you listen to your body, it will to you when you need food and when you don't.

Luckily, all of the steps to changing how you eat work together. By recognizing your motives for eating, you will naturally start listening to your body. By slowing down and taking the time to eat, you will naturally start consuming smaller portion sizes. Each step builds on the other to help you cultivate a healthier relationship with food.

Educate yourself about food

Once you have started to change how you eat, you can begin the process of changing what you eat. However, in order to do so, you must be educated about food. Be passionate about the food that goes in your body!

Let's start with the defining the basics of any healthy diet: protein, carbohydrates, fats, and vitamins and minerals.

Protein: The body uses protein to grow, repair, or replace tissue. Protein is also involved in producing enzymes, hormones, and antibodies. It is needed for blood clotting and maintaining the body's fluid balance (among other important functions). Protein is made up of amino acids. There are 22 amino acids that are considered vital to your health; but the human body can only make 14 of these 22. The other eight must be obtained from food. This is where protein comes in!

Protein can be found in all kinds of food, but only fish, meat, eggs, cheese, and other foods that come from animal sources contain complete proteins and supply the necessary eight amino acids. You should always seek lean sources of protein.

Carbohydrates: Carbohydrates, along with fats, provide the lion's share of the fuel your body needs. Both of these macronutrients are broken down into glucose: the body's primary energy source. Glucose provides nearly all the energy your brain uses each day. Or they may be converted in glycogen, which is how energy is stored. These stores must be replenished or the body's protein is dismantled to make glucose. Carbohydrates are the only dietary source of fiber. The best sources of carbohydrates are those with little or no fat, such as vegetables, fruits legumes, and grains.

Fats: Fats are necessary for good health. Fats provide fat-soluble vitamins (vitamins A, D, E & K, for those of you with a burning desire to know). They're needed to regulate hormones and to contribute structure to our cells. They help keep the body warm and protect it from mechanical shock. They slow digestion and provide a sense of satiety so that you don't keep feeling hungry after eating. Fats can be mono- unsaturated, poly-unsaturated, saturated, and trans fat. Mono-unsaturated fats are the "good" fats found in olive oil, nuts, avocado, etc. Trans fat and saturated fat are the most unhealthy forms of fat. Studies show that diets rich in saturated fat can contribute to high cholesterol, increased risk of heart disease, and increased risk of certain types of cancer.

Vitamins and minerals: Vitamins and minerals are natural substances contained in a wide variety of foods that have long been recognized as essential to maintaining healthy body systems. You must get your vitamins and minerals from food; your body does not produce them. Scientists have defined specific daily amounts of vitamins and minerals that are necessary for good health.

Now that you understand that basics, it's time to take a closer look at "good food" versus "bad food." Good food promotes health and prevents disease—it lubricates your arteries and increases your energy level. Bad food, however, can increase your risk for disease: it can clog your arteries and negatively affect your body's basic functions. Before we dive into the truth of unhealthy foods, remember that my goal is not to scare you! Ultimately, it is *your* decision to choose what foods you put into your body. What's more, any healthy and balanced diet will include some of everything—both the good and the bad. The key is to be sensible with your choices.

When it comes to confusion about food, the greatest challenge for most Americans falls in two clear areas: **fat** and **carbohydrates**. Above all else, if you can figure out how to eat more of the good fat and more of the good carbohydrates, you'll be well on your way to lifelong health.

Fat—the good, bad, and ugly
We all know that fat can be bad. In fact, must Americans fear fat and avoid it at all costs. But despite what you may think, **we need fat** in our daily diet. Fats keep your skin soft, give you energy, and make your cells flexible and elastic. Many vitamins are more readily available when eaten with fat. Most importantly, fats from food provide the body with essential fatty acids that contribute to overall health and disease prevention. Avoiding fat altogether is not only unrealistic, it's also unhealthy. You don't need a "low-fat diet," you need a "good fat" diet: the key is knowing the difference.

Let's start with the good guys—unsaturated fats—which are derived from plants. Unsaturated fat comes in two forms, monounsaturated and polyunsaturated, both of which help lower your bad (LDL) cholesterol and raise your good (HDL) cholesterol. Polyunsaturated fat is particularly good because it supplies the body with omega-3 fatty acids, which have been shown to contribute to the construction of cell membranes. Numerous research studies indicate that a diet high in omega-3 fatty acid is associated with reductions in heart attacks and strokes, lowered cholesterol and triglycerides levels, and a lower risk of hypertension. In addition, omega-3 fatty acids tend to suppress inflammation.

Here are the main differences in unsaturated fat:

- **Monounsaturated fat** remains liquid at room temperature but may start to solidify in the refrigerator. Foods high in monounsaturated fat include olive, peanut, and canola oils. Avocados and most nuts also have high amounts of monounsaturated fat. Canola and Olive oil are the only fats you should have in the pantry. Don't fry but sauté is the word of the future. Monounsaturated fats have advantages and there does not appear to be a link between them and a high risk of colon, breast and prostate cancer.

- **Polyunsaturated fat** is usually liquid at room temperature and in the refrigerator. Foods high in polyunsaturated fats include vegetable oils such as safflower, corn, sunflower, soy, and cottonseed oils. These fats lower cholesterol but may increase cancer risk.

- **Omega-3 fatty acids** are polyunsaturated fats found mostly in seafood and in many nuts. Good sources of omega-3s include fatty cold-water fish such as salmon, mackerel, and herring. Flaxseeds, flax oil, and walnuts also contain omega-3 fatty acids, and small amounts are found in soybean and canola oils.

Think of unsaturated fat as the superheroes of the fat world. They are the nutrients that actually help your body promote health and prevent disease. But no superhero would be complete without its villain counterpart. So now let's move on to the more dangerous denizens of the fat world: saturated fat and trans fat.

Saturated fat is decidedly less healthy than unsaturated fat. Typically found in animal sources such as butter, meat, eggs, and cheese, saturated fat can be directly linked to increased levels of cholesterol. It can also be found in coconut oil and palm oil. Saturated fat also contains essential fatty acids, primarily omega-6 fatty acid. Omega-6 fatty acid is a vital component to a healthy diet; however, most Americans get far too much of. If the body contains too much saturated fat or too high concentrations of omega-6 fatty acids, the cell membranes are less elastic. In heart vessels, less elastic vessels predispose to the accumulation of fat that leads to heart attacks and strokes.

Ultimately, a little saturated fat in your daily diet is not a problem—but a *lot* of saturated fat certainly is. When it comes to saturated fat, the key is moderation.

The biggest villain in the fat world by far is trans fat. You should avoid trans fat at all costs. Trans fat, also known as trans fatty acids, is a man-made form of fat used to prolong a product's shelf-life. These fats form when vegetable oil hardens through a process called hydrogenation. Trans fat actually raise bad cholesterol and lower good cholesterol, the exactly opposite effect of unsaturated fats. They are found in fried foods, commercial baked goods, processed foods, and margarine. Whenever you see "hydrogenated" or "partially hydrogenated" on a product's label, don't eat it.

Good carbs vs. bad carbs (complex vs. simple)
Ever since the outbreak of the Atkins diet, Americans have feared carbohydrates. This is such a shame, because carbohydrates are fantastic and necessary nutrients for any healthy diet. But like fats, there are good carbs and bad carbs.

When it comes to carbohydrates, the key is the glycemic index. The glycemic index is a tool used to rank carbohydrates by how quickly each food source turns to sugar in your body. Carbohydrates that turn to glucose very slowly are complex carbohydrates. These are the foods that fuel the body with long-lasting energy, improve digestion, decrease hunger, and lower the risk of many common illnesses. Complex carbohydrates are found in whole grains, vegetables, legumes, and certain cereals, which offer a full array of nutritional benefits. Simple carbohydrates, however, quickly convert to sugar in the body, offer little nutritional value and contribute to higher incidence of diabetes. Simple carbohydrates are found in fruit, juice, sugar, and many processed foods. The glycemic index ranks carbohydrate sources on a scale of 0 to 100. Your most complex carbs have low GI ratings, while simple carbs rank very high.

Thankfully, the glycemic index demystifies the whole process of how to choose good carbs over bad ones. For example, a baked Russet potato ranks 100 on the glycemic index, while a baked sweet potato ranks 60. So if you're looking to have a baked potato for dinner, choose a sweet potato over a regular white potato. Remember, eliminate the idea that carbohydrates are only found in bread! Carbohydrates are in juice, candy, fruit, crackers, salad dressing, beans, nuts, and the list goes on and on. Learn to read labels and empower yourself to decipher exactly what kind of carbohydrates you're consuming. The glycemic index will certainly help, but over time you should be able to guess whether it's a good carb or a bad carb, complex or simple.

#1 Tool in your health arsenal: label reading

Perhaps the #1 tool in your health arsenal is learning to read labels. Just take a walk down your supermarket aisle and notice how many products claim to be "natural" or "fresh" or "additive-free." There is no regulation on these terms, so it doesn't necessarily mean that the food is healthy. There can be such a huge variance in the claims that it's absolutely imperative that you know how to read nutritional labels. This is only way truly to understand what you're eating. So, here's a quick crash course:

Here is the most essential information:

Calories. *The first thing to look for on a label is the amount of calories per serving. Be aware if the product is extremely high in calories.*

Serving size and number of servings per container. *This information is critical to understanding everything else on the label. The number of calories may not look too high, until you realize that there are four servings per container! Be sure to account for the fact that you may not typically consume the recommended serving size.*

Dietary Fiber. *Look for foods that are high in fiber. To be considered high in fiber, a food must contain at least five grams per serving.*

Fat. *Now that manufacturers to show the fat makeup of each product, it's considerably easier to choose the good, unsaturated fats over the foods with saturated and trans fats (also called trans fatty acids).*

Sodium per serving. *Sodium should be restricted to 2,300 mg per day (that's less than 1 teaspoon of salt) for healthy adults, and 1,500 mg for those with health problems or family histories of high blood pressure.*

Sugar. *Sugar is a simple carbohydrate that adds plenty of calories to your foods. Remember that four grams of sugar is equal to one teaspoon.*

% Daily value (% DV). This is based on a 2,000-calorie diet and reflects the percentage of a certain nutrient that the food supplies. It gives you a rough idea of the food's nutrient contribution to your diet.

Ingredient list. Manufacturers are required to list all of the ingredients contained in the product by weight. The first ingredient listed is the most prevalent ingredient in the food. So, if the first ingredient is "high fructose corn syrup," that means that sugar is the main ingredient and you should likely limit your intake.

Nutrition Facts

Serving Size 3 oz. (85g)

Amount Per Serving

Calories 38   **Calories from Fat** 0

	% Daily Value*
Total Fat 0g	0%
Saturated Fat 0g	0%
Cholesterol 0g	0%
Sodium 0g	2%
Total Carbohydrate 0g	3%
Dietary Fiber 0g	8%
Sugars 0g	
Protein 0g	
Vitamin A	270%
Calcium	2%
Vitamin C	10%
Iron	0%

*Percent Daily Values are based on a 2,000 calorie diet. Your daily values may be higher or lower depending on your calorie needs:

	Calories:	2,000	2,500
Total Fat	Less than	65g	80g
Sat Fat	Less than	20g	80g
Cholesterol	Less than	300mg	300mg
Sodium	Less than	2,400mg	2,400mg
Total Carbohydrate		300g	375g
Dietary Fiber		25g	30g

The final note
There is one final note on developing a healthy relationship with food: **find your body's natural weight and be happy with it.** This is such an overlooked and misunderstood element of weight loss. If you incorporate all of these steps to living a healthy life—eating more of the right foods, for the right reasons, and in the right way— your body will find its own healthy weight. We are not all meant to be the same size and dimension. Some of us are big on top, small on bottom, skinny all around. It does not matter. Your image is not the main focus. You cannot develop a healthy relationship with food, without simultaneously cultivating a healthy relationship with your body image. A key component of living a healthy life is learning to accept who you are and what you look like. When it comes to food, passion is found when you free yourself from the emotional burden of trying to look like someone else.

Putting it all together

By now you have learned how to free yourself from diets and de- velop a healthy relationship with food. The final challenge is to put it all together and actually implement changes into your daily life. Most people think that this final step is the most difficult to master. Truthfully, every other weight-loss book and nutrition bible feed in to that idea. You could spend years reading through each different prescription for exactly what to eat. The weight-loss industry has made millions convincing people that there is one specific path to healthy eating. And each new author on the market seems to bring a new plan and a new prescription. No wonder Americans are confused about how to eat well! For me, it has become way too complicated.

My goal in teaching anyone how to eat well is to empower him or her to make healthy choices. There are millions of healthy choices out there—not just boring or seemingly "healthy" salads! If you change how you eat and educate yourself about food, the wide array of healthy eating becomes so clear. Believe me, learning to develop a healthy relationship with food is a much more difficult task than actually putting the "right" food on your plate.

For me, it's imperative that we simplify the process of creating a healthy diet. We all know that your body needs a combination of protein, carbohydrates, fats, vitamins, and minerals. With a little research, you can find very clear prescriptions on exactly how much of each category you should consume. No more than 20 grams of this or no more than 40% of that. Although these statistics may be true, they just don't speak to me. When it comes to choosing my food, the sterility of numbers and percentages is just too off-putting. I am passionate about my food … not about ensuring I get the perfect ratio of protein to fat!

I approach healthy eating with two main points in mind: 1) there is a wide path to promoting health and preventing disease and 2) some foods are worth being passionate about.

Find *your* path to healthy eating: ReCenter your plate
You have a lot of freedom in developing your own path to healthy eating. You may like some foods more than others. Or you may have a particular weakness for chocolate or cheese. Whatever it is, there is a way for you to create a healthy diet.

In order to convey this freedom, I like to use the ReCenter Food Target. This is something my daughter created through a health-promotion program called ReCenter. But I'll steal it from her for a moment! The ReCenter Food Target is meant to help you navigate the daily decisions of what to eat. All foods fall somewhere on this target. Healthy eating should be simple: aim for the center of the target, and eat *more* of these foods. Venture out into the outer rings and limit your intake.

Remember that passion is not likely found in a narrow interpretation of living a healthy life! There is a wide path to healthy eating. Let the food target serve as a guide on this path. Here it is:

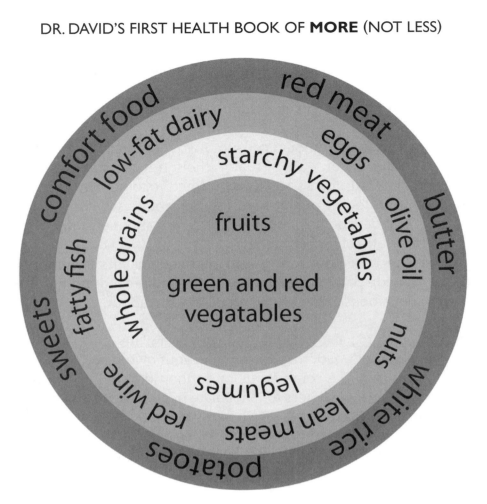

If you are completely new to healthy eating or if you must lose weight for health reasons, stick to the center of the target. Don't cut out whole categories of foods or skip a meal to reduce your daily calories. Chances are these strategies won't work. Feeling deprived of your favorite foods, or not eating a meal altogether, could lead to overeating later on. Instead, fuel your body throughout the day mostly with vegetables, fruits, whole grains, and beans. Consider this the beginning of a life-changing process. Stay with a narrow selection of healthy foods and re-orient your body to a new way of eating. Eat limited amounts of foods within the blue circle and completely avoid anything in the red, outer ring. Always remember to pay attention to serving size!

If you understand the basics of healthy eating and currently practice some elements of good nutrition, your path to lifelong nutrition is somewhat wider. You have more leeway to navigate throughout the green, yellow, and blue rings. However, you must continue to develop proper eating habits. You do not yet have free reign to the whole gamut of foods. Avoid fatty foods, cook in a healthful way, and use sugars sparingly. Falling in this middle category of eating forces more personal accountability and tests your understanding of good nutrition.

Finally, if you have totally mastered the art of healthy eating, you have free reign to adopt the widest path of nutrition. Use the food target as a loose guide. Eat the "right" foods and fuel your body with nutrition-packed meals. You'll feel better, look better, and live better.

Eight foods I'm passionate about

There is a huge array of foods that promote health and prevent disease. While you must launch your own personal quest to develop a healthy diet, I'd like to offer up the foods that I am most passionate about as a starting point.

Remember that the best way to get healthful nutrients, rich in vitamins, minerals, and antioxidants comes from a natural diet—not from liquid supplements, nutritional extracts, tablets or capsules. Antioxidant pills do not prolong life, prevent cancer, or reduce the risk of heart attacks and strokes but a diet rich in antioxidants does.

1. Olive oil

1 to 2 tablespoons a day

High in omega-3 fatty acids and Vitamin E, olive oil is a great protector of the heart. Olive oil is full of the "right fats"—monounsaturated and polyunsaturated fats that have been shown to improve blood flow, maintain elasticity in the veins, and "lube" the heart as it ages. Its healthful properties abound, protecting the heart against disease and reducing blood pressure. I try to stick to one to two tablespoons of olive oil a day. If you cannot use olive oil while cooking, try canola or sunflower oil (which are also high in omega-3 fatty acids).

2. Fruits and vegetables
As much as you want!
The average American woefully underestimates the power of fruits and vegetables. Filled with vitamins and nutrients, fruits and vegetables fuel the body with energy and protect you against disease. You can eat as many fruits and vegetables you want. Remember, when you choose your foods, strive to get the full spectrum of colors. Deeply hued fruits and vegetables provide the wide range of vitamins, minerals, fiber, and phytochemicals your body needs to maintain good health and energy levels, protect against disease, and reduce the risk of cancer. Always try to eat whole fruit rather than fruit juice! It offers much more nutritional power.

3. Whole grains
5 to 6 servings a day
Rich in complex carbohydrates, whole grains are made up of starches and soluble and insoluble fiber. I try to consume around six servings of whole grains per day. Since unrefined carbs provide fiber, they help control hunger by making you feel full. Additionally, diets high in dietary fiber may moderate blood sugar in diabetics and blood cholesterol levels for anyone, and contain cancer-fighting vitamins and phytochemicals.

4. Lean meats
3 to 4 ounces twice a day
Protein powers the body with sustaining and energizing fuel. Your body needs low-fat forms of protein every day. Lean meats such as turkey, chicken, wild game, venison, and low-fat cuts of pork and beef fuel the body with necessary protein while still avoiding saturated fat. Lean meats also contain healthy levels of Omega-3 and Omega-6 fatty acids.

5. Fatty fish

4 to 6 ounces twice a week

Fatty, cold-water fish, including salmon, trout, sardines, and albacore tuna contain high levels of omega-3 fatty acids. Studies show that consumption of EPA (eicosapentaenoic acid) and DHA (docosahexaenoic acid) omega-3 fatty acids reduce the risk of coronary artery disease, lower triglycerides, lower cholesterol, reduce the risk of depression, and reduce the risk of breast and colon cancer. The American Heart Association recommends that everyone consume fish twice weekly, with a strong emphasis on fatty fish.

6. Nuts

A handful a day

Nuts are concentrated sources of plant protein, which are chock-full of heart-healthy mono-unsaturated fatty acids, vitamins, and minerals. Roasted or raw, nuts have a variety of textures and tastes, adding great variety to your palate. Remember, a handful of nuts per day can reduce your risk of heart disease. However, eight handfuls will not. Always consume nuts in moderation!

> **Walnuts.** My first choice for alpha-linolenic acid (ALA), walnuts are incredibly heart-healthy. Their rich nutritional content helps prevent cardiovascular disease.

> **Almonds.** Prized as a premier natural source of vitamin E, almonds are rich in protein, iron, riboflavin, and magnesium. While almonds have a lower fat content than other nuts, they still prove a good source of monounsaturated fats.

7. Wine

1-2 glasses a day

Rich in flavonoids and anti-oxidants, red wine in moderation protects the heart against disease and increases levels of (good) HDL cholesterol. A staple of the Mediterranean diet, a glass of red wine twice daily has been proven to protect the heart and the brain, reducing the risk of Alzheimer's disease. Remember, always drink in moderation!

More than two glasses per day is not only bad for your health, but also dangerous.
As you age, your body becomes more susceptible to liver damage from excess alcohol

8. Chocolate
Twice a week
After much research, scientists now believe a little dark chocolate each day actually improves your health and prevents disease! While this remains a debatable topic, one thing is true—a little dessert is lovely. Dessert can range from fruit and cheese to cookies and ice cream. Desserts offer a nice end to a healthy meal or a tiny splurge after a long week.

No matter what your personal vice, desserts deserve attention. So don't be afraid to splurge a little. Be passionate about your food and let a little chocolate liven up your life.

Putting passion back in your diet: *more* food, not less.
Eating a good meal is perhaps one of my greatest joys in life. I can truly appreciate beautiful food, whether or not it's one-hundred-percent healthy. I think this is the greatest lesson every American should learn. Food deserves to be respected and enjoyed! Stop stressing about every little morsel that passes your lips and rather choose to develop a healthy relationship with your food. If you are educated about your health, making the right choices is simple. What's more, there is no need to adhere to some ridiculously strict prescription for healthful meals. Find balance in everything—from butter and wine, to spinach and walnuts!

Nutrition is a key component of living a healthy life, but it is only one part of a more comprehensive plan. Diets never work and weight loss is not the goal.

CHAPTER 9
MORE MOVEMENT

Though you may not know it, scientists have already found the one magic bullet that will prolong life, prevent disease, and ensure life-long independence. It's not sexy, nor is it groundbreaking. It's easy and hard, simple and complex all at the same time. It's exercise.

Exercise, at any age, is the best life insurance policy you could ever buy. Whether you start early or late, the benefits of moving more are astounding. Unfortunately, Americans hate to exercise. Believe me, I have heard every excuse in the book. It's too hard, I'm too old, I'm too tired, I'm too busy. When it comes to exercise, the excuses abound.

Enticing Americans to exercise can be a challenging task, so in the last five years the medical community has rallied around one single mantra: "Just do a little. Anything is better than nothing." While any exercise is better than no exercise, the idea that less is more is simply wrong! This passive, mediocre approach not only provides yet another excuse for us to avoid the hard work of healthy living, but also sucks the life out of exercising! Where is the passion in a leisurely, 10-minute stroll? You don't even give your body a chance to release the healthy, energizing endorphins of exercise.

When it comes to exercise, throw age out the window. Don't slow down after 50—speed up! It's even more important now that you keep up the momentum and make exercise a part of your daily life.

The eighth step in Dr. David's Longevity plan is *more* movement. Get off your butt and make fitness a priority. Move more, not less as you age. Whether you're 45, 55, or 85, the benefits of an effective and appropriate exercise regimen are astounding.

The Lipschitz way
Let me first say that the Lipschitz clan is not filled with athletes. At six-foot-three, I'm clumsy and pigeon-toed. A run around the block is simply not in the cards. What's more, I do not exactly have

145

a fitness-friendly family. I recently suggested to my mother that she might want to set aside a little time for regular exercise. She looked at me and said, "Oy vay, David, you are killing me. When I get the urge to exercise, I lie down and stay there until the urge goes away." Suffice it to say that I am not Lance Armstrong or Jack LaLanne. I don't exercise for hours on end and I certainly don't have a body fat percentage in the teens!

You do not have be a crazy exercise nut to be fit. Fitness does not necessarily mean training for the Tour de France or completing an Ironman at 55. A six-pack of abs and bulging biceps is not the litmus test of fitness. Although both of those challenges are incredible for sure, often we psych ourselves out thinking that a rigorous exercise program is limited to hard-core athletes. This is simply not true. You do not have to stick to some idealized image of what it means to be "in shape." Fitness comes in all shapes, sizes and forms.

When I was in my early 30s, jogging was the craze. Like many of my friends, I decided to take it up. I never enjoyed it, nor did I ever experience the so-called "runner's high." But four times a week for five years, I religiously pounded the pavements for three miles. I can still see myself, a lumbering elephant, struggling up mild inclines with a frown on my face. Shin splints, joint pains, and the occasional twilight tumble plagued my foray into fitness. It was horrible! When it came to running, I was the opposite of passionate. After awhile, I found myself coming up with any excuse to skip my daily run. Finally, I stopped altogether.

At the time, I had all sorts of explanations as to why exercise wasn't working for me. But several years later—unfit and overweight—my body simply couldn't keep up and the mild heart attack I experienced was the last wake-up call I'll ever need to start exercising again. From that day on, my commitment to improve my health never faltered. I kept telling myself the same thing I told my 80 year old patients: "It's never too early, or too late, to start exercising." Jogging clearly wouldn't work, so I launched a journey to find the right exercise program for me. When I discovered the joy of indoor bikes, my life forever changed. I watch TV while

I pedal away, and the time flashes by. I also found that brisk walking worked my heart as well as running but without the physical and mental anguish!

It took a long time, but I finally found my own exercise niche. Today, I alternate indoor biking with one-hour walks and I resistance-train at a gym two to three times weekly. Lance Armstrong could kick my butt, but I've never felt better.

If I can exercise, anyone can. My story is simply one example of how fitness comes in many forms. My method for staying fit might not be yours, but the goal is to find any avenue to exercise and tap in to the healing qualities of fitness.

Exercise and your health

Beyond my own personal anecdotes and experiences, it's hard to miss the compelling evidence that exercise adds years to your life. Research consistently shows that fitness, both aerobic and strength training, promote health and prevent diseases across the spectrum.

Exercise assists your body work at its optimum level. With cardiovascular training, you work the most important muscle in your body—your heart. A stronger heart means fewer heart attacks and more blood pumping through the body with less exertion. This, in turn, lowers your blood pressure and reduces the risk of strokes. Regular exercise helps your body regulate excess weight and speeds up your metabolism. It also reduces your risk of diabetes, colon cancer, breast cancer, osteoporosis, prostate cancer and depression.

Simply put, exercise helps to improve virtually every bodily function!

Because regular exercise promotes health and prevents disease, the link to longevity is obvious. If you prevent diseases and maintain a healthy, well-functioning body, you will live longer.

An aging body needs exercise

Let's get back to the basics of *why* your body needs exercise. First, it's important to understand how your body changes with time.

Between the ages of 20 and 60, the average individual gains about a pound a year. This weight gain is accompanied by one of the most predictable features of growing older, loss of muscle and increase in fat. At age 20, the average thigh is over 90% muscle and 10% fat. But by age 60, the ratio of muscle to fat drops to 50:50. By the time many adults reach their 80th birthday, they will have lost more than 50% of their peak muscle mass.

Just look at the following illustration. It is a CAT scan of 20-year-old woman's thigh compared to one of a quite fit and healthy 63-year-old woman. The dark area is muscle and the white is fat. The image says it all.

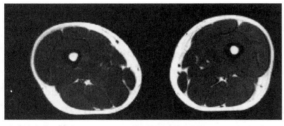

A CAT scan of
the thigh of a
20-year-old woman

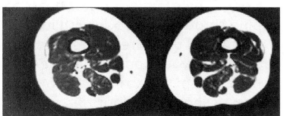

A CAT scan of
the thigh of a
63-year-old woman

My colleague, Dr. William Evans, is the leading authority on how age affects muscle strength and function. He was the first to coin the now widely used term, "sarcopenia," which describes the loss of muscle with age. Dr. Evans found that there are two kinds of muscle fibers, fast twitch and slow twitch, and they diminish at different stages of life. Fast twitch is primarily used for sprinting and jumping, while slow twitch is essential for long distance walking or running. Beginning at age 20, the fast twitch muscle begins to disappear while the slow twitch declines much later. This is why the world's fastest sprinters peak before the age of 25, yet the leading marathoners run best in their 30s.

Ultimately, for sprinters, marathoners, and everyone else, this loss of muscle leads to a significant loss of strength, which—without treatment—can have grave effects on an aging body. Only recently have we begun to understand the root cause of age-related muscle loss. Scientists discovered that primitive muscle cells called myoblasts proliferate as muscle fibers diminish. Myoblasts mature into cells called myocytes, which repair damaged muscles and replace muscle fibers that have been destroyed by injuries.

The ability of myocytes to repair muscle appears to diminish over time. In addition, there's some evidence that an older person's myoblasts, rather than maturing into muscle-building myocytes, get "diverted" and form more fat cells. These effects are in full swing by age 50 and continue with advancing age.

We're still not sure what reduces the ability of myocytes to function normally. Genetic changes might be involved. It could also be due to decades of exposure to oxidants and free radicals, byproducts of metabolism that damage cells throughout the body. As we learn more about the things that damage myocytes, we may someday be able to manipulate the genetic composition of myoblasts, make them young again, and perhaps prevent age-related muscle declines. But for now, the only way to build muscle tissue is with exercise. Without it, Mother Nature seems to work against you.

Most people become more sedentary with age. Though it often begins with seemingly benign and natural "slowing down," becoming sedentary in your 50s or 60s can lead to a very nasty downward spiral by your 70s or 80s. Remaining sedentary and failing to reverse the progressive loss of muscle has profound implications.

Muscles that aren't worked get progressively weaker, which reduces your body's ability to maintain the integrity of joints. Combined with normal wear and tear, this can lead to osteoarthritis, the most common chronic medical problem after age 50. Joint pain is often the reason we stop running, playing tennis, or even walking. Thus begins a terrible cycle. Unused muscles keep getting weaker.

Weak muscles fail to support the joints. The joints get increasingly stiff and painful, so we exercise even less.

Muscle weakness is also a direct cause of age-related bone loss, or osteoporosis, which affects millions of older adults. Though men can get osteoporosis, it's more common in women. After menopause, the bones can get so weak that they spontaneously fracture. Even if the bones hold together, osteoporosis is a major cause of aches and pains, as well as significant disability.

Once you're sedentary and weak—regardless of the cause—the risk of falls and fractures increases. Fracturing a major bone is often disastrous and can lead to permanent disability, physical dependence, and a high risk of early death. If you are over the age of 75 and break a hip, there is 50% chance you will never walk normally again. What's more, there is a good chance you will be admitted to a nursing home and die within one year. The vast majority of these complications could be prevented with regular, vigorous exercise.

It is impossible to stop the loss of muscle with age. Nor is it possible to turn 80-year-old bones into the bones of a teenage athlete. What we can do, however, is make the bones stronger. We can build muscle to support older joints. We can increase flexibility, improve balance, build strength, increase circulation and prevent virtually all of the negative effects of an aging body … all with exercise.

Exercise in the obesity era

Although the data is clear and exercise is nature's very best "longevity pill," Americans hate to exercise. We are not exactly a nation of movers—instead, we're drivers, sitters, and eaters. The average community has expanded to such an extent that it's impossible to walk anywhere. The neighborhood grocery store is almost extinct, and even if you do live in a pedestrian friendly area, Americans are more likely to drive even a short mile to get to the local coffee shop. Many of us spend the majority of the day sitting at work, at home, or in the car. The "exercise culture" is definitely not the mainstream, and rather relegated to an "athlete culture" where fitness is a 24-hour pursuit!

However, as our waistlines continue to expand and the implications for an unhealthy nation grow, the medical community (along with great help from the mainstream media) has pushed Americans to focus on living a healthy lifestyle. In order to entice us to relinquish the sedentary living, the "powers that be" have tried to spread the message that a little exercise is all you need and it's just as good as a lot of exercise. They dumbed-down the exercise prescription, pitching it as a necessary evil rather than a passionate pursuit.

I'm not entirely sure how the "less is more" approach to exercise got started. Yes, modest amounts of exercise can promote weight loss and reduce the risk of diabetes and heart disease. Some exercise is better than no exercise. But it hardly follows that some exercise is just as good as *more* exercise.

The tendency to view exercise as a necessary evil has only increased in the wake of recent reports that suggest people can get dramatic health gains with minimal exertion, such as walking at a snail's pace for half an hour a day. Even better, they say you don't need to exercise for prolonged amounts of time! You can complete your entire exercise regimen "easy, 10-minute sessions." With that kind of advice floating around the scientific community and in the mainstream media, it's hardly surprising that people have hung up their tennis rackets and hauled the treadmill to a forgotten corner in the basement. Why get all tired and sweaty if a leisurely stroll around the block provides the same benefits?

Unfortunately, many of my patients have taken these messages to heart. They're convinced that strolling a couple times a day will provide the same benefits as sweating through a tough exercise session. I have to say that the medical community is complicit in this unintentional ruse. Americans, on average, get so little exercise and are so out of shape that my colleagues and I are thrilled if we can get them to do anything more vigorous than walking to the refrigerator. A doctor who convinces a sedentary patient to commit to a walking program, even if it's only for half an hour three times a week, will feel a little glow of victory. But that much exercise, frankly, is nowhere near enough.

Fit and fat?
So here is the dilemma: In the past 10 years, we have gotten progressively fatter and less active. But which is more important? The pounds or the activity?

In *More Food* (chapter seven), I discussed the evidence that being overweight is associated with a longer life expectancy. This particularly applies to anyone over the age of 70 where weight loss, either voluntary or involuntary, is associated with an increased risk of illness and death. Ultimately, I think the health-care community and diet industry have overstated the impact of American's growing girth. Losing weight to "get into shape" or fit someone else's ideal body type is never a good idea. However, as with most things in health, the relationship with weight and longevity is nuanced and complex. Extra pounds may help you live longer, but this is not the same as living *better*.

After the age of 60, the combined effect of less muscle and more fat makes overweight individuals at a much greater risk of weakness, frailty and difficulty walking. There is a very important message here. Being pleasantly plump is clearly associated with a longer but not a **better** life expectancy. Being plump and sedentary is a prescription for physical disability, problems with gait and balance and an inability to live alone. But combine being plump with exercise and your future can be bright.

It *is* possible to be fit and fat. In fact, if you are fat, you'd better be fit! All it takes is regular exercise and a chubby person can remain as physically strong or stronger than any sedentary peer, thin or not. Research done at the Cooper clinic has clearly shown that overweight individuals who exercise are far healthier than sedentary individuals who are thin. Furthermore, overweight individuals who still exercise have a significantly lower risk of heart disease and stroke than someone who looks to be "in good shape" but doesn't exercise. The trends over the last 20 years suggest that it's the lack of exercise, as much as diet, that's responsible for the dramatic rise of obesity. In the years 1980 to 1991, a time when the prevalence of obesity was surging, the average calorie intake actually declined from 1850 to 1780 per day. At the same time, total fat intake decreased by 11%. So the reason we're getting fat is *not* because we're eating more, but because we're not exercising.

And yet for the overweight and unfit among us, the first thing everyone says is "lose weight." Unfortunately, that saying is almost always associated with dieting rather than exercise. But this is not a message about weight: it's a message about fitness. For every pound of fat lost by dieting, a pound of muscle is lost as well. Dieting leads to a higher risk of illness and death. If the diet fails and the weight returns, it is all in the form of fat with virtually no return of the lost muscle. This leads to even more weakness, a greater risk of falling and an even higher risk of further disability.

In the longevity game, fitness trumps nutrition every time. If you are overweight, the message is simple: exercise first and then tackle any issues with your diet.

How much exercise? How vigorous?
So how much exercise do people really need? Is walking two miles a day enough for those 60 years and older? What about adults in their 40s and 50s?

I get asked these questions all the time, and my answer is always the same: Get more. If you currently exercise for 20 minutes at a time, increase it to 30 or 40 minutes. If you enjoy slow walking, pick up the pace and walk briskly. Increasing the time that you exercise, or exercising more intensely, will elevate your exercise tolerance. The better your maximum exercise tolerance, the longer you're going to live.

The research supports this philosophy. In 2007 researchers from the University of Pittsburgh showed that the more briskly and the longer an individual walks, the greater the benefit on life expectancy. A study conducted in Great Britain in 1995 claimed that moderate to mild exercise had no major health benefits. Researchers examined the impact of vigorous exercise on longevity in over 9000 civil servants ranging in age from 45 to 64. The subjects were divided into two groups: one group exercised vigorously while the other group participated in non-vigorous activities. Vigorous activity included jogging, swimming, tennis, football, hockey, hiking, and football. Non-vigorous exercise included golf, dancing, and table tennis.

The benefits varied depending on the age of the men. Between the ages of 45 and 54, vigorous exercisers who exercised twice a week had a 67% reduction in the risk of a heart attack and an 80% reduction in the risk of dying. Those who exercised less strenuously or fewer times per week experienced dramatically lower benefits.

However, the results were somewhat different for slightly older men between the ages of 55 and 64. For this generation, smaller amounts of high intensity exercise seemed very beneficial. Vigorous exercise completed as little as one to three times per month lowered heart attack risk by 25%. Vigorous exercise once weekly lowered the risk by 50% and twice weekly by 65%. These statistics also correlated with a lower risk of death.

In this study, men of any age who completed mild to moderate exercise received no quantitative health benefits. So if all you did was prune the fence, ride the golf cart between holes, or take a stroll around the block, your risk of heart attack or an earlier death was not affected.

Another study, however, focused on the benefits of low-intensity physical activity. Originally published in the *New England Journal of Medicine* in 2002, this study examined the effect of moderate exercise for retired non-smoking men. Those who walked regularly lived longer than those who didn't walk at all. However, the men who walked less than a mile a day had twice the mortality rates of those who walked more than two miles! By any reasonable standards, a two-mile walk for a man in his 70s or 80s is a hefty workout. In this instance, low-impact may not be the same as low-intensity: what is easy for one person may not be for another.

In 2007, researchers from Harvard Medical school released data from the 10-year Women's Health Initiative that showed moderate exercise reduced the risk of heart disease by 27 to 41%. All of the 27,055 participants were women working in health care who, between the years 1995 and 1999, were free of either cancer or any evidence of heart disease. Over a 10-year period, 979 of the women developed heart problems. For the women walked two hours a week, the risk of developing heart disease was noticeably lower.

As you can see, the studies and the data vary. It's difficult to determine the exact amount of exercise necessary to obtain quantitative health benefits. However, one thing is clear: when you do exercise, it should be challenging. If you push yourself, raise your heart rate, challenge your muscles, and expand your lungs, the corresponding health benefits will come. Unfortunately, less than 20% of Americans exercise strenuously. In fact, approximately 24% of the population over the age of 64 is totally inactive. That's a health bomb waiting to go off!

The "toos"

Researchers have spent a great amount of time investigating why we don't exercise. How can an activity that is so clearly beneficial be viewed with so much disdain? The most obvious and easiest reasons are genetic and physiological factors. Some people may be genetically predisposed to have good flexibility, balance, and strength. Some people are "natural athletes." Others—like me—are more clumsy or not as well-built. But frankly, these are ridiculous cop-outs!

People always have reasons why getting regular exercise is flat-out impossible. I've found that these reasons usually involve the word "too." I am too busy, too tired, too sick, too old, too weak, too fat, or too intimidated. Let's take a look at the most common exercise excuses:

I'm too busy. This one never holds up very well. Everyone can get a thoroughly vigorous workout in 20 to 30 minutes. If you're really so busy that you can't set aside half an hour a day, than your priorities need adjusting. Get up half an hour earlier in the morning. Give up the evening news. Forget the afternoon nap. Whatever it takes, set aside the time to exercise. People who are truly so busy that they can't find time to exercise are looking at a grim future.

In my experience, people who say they're too busy to exercise are really saying that they're too stressed. That by itself is going to lead to illness. But exercise is a natural stress reliever! Remember all the pent up energy that your body produces during a "fight or flight" response? You release it during exercise! Exercise actually allows your body to come down to a more regulated state. You'll feel better, function better, and enjoy life more. To top it off, exercise boosts energy and productivity—making you more efficient and productive in your non-exercising hours.

I'm too tired. The too tired excuse often goes hand in hand with "too busy" and "too stressed." One of the best ways to treat fatigue is to exercise. Exercise improves metabolism and promotes better sleep. It also stimulates the release of hormones and cytokines, natural chemicals that promote feelings of energy and well-being. Fatigue is usually caused by stress, poor sleep, depression, some medications, or illness. Don't ignore fatigue, especially if it's so pronounced that you feel you can't exercise because of it. Talk to your doctor and come up with a solution.

I'm too sick. Obviously, I wouldn't advise anyone with a bad cold to jog three miles on an icy morning. But what if you have a long-term illness such as severe arthritis, cancer, or heart disease? The evidence is compelling that exercise is important in the recovery of every major disease. A study of patients with osteoarthritis, for example, showed that intensive exercise, both aerobic and resistance training, significantly reduced symptoms and disability. Exercise is also an integral part of rehabilitation following a heart attack or open-heart surgery. In fact, people who take up an exercise program are three times less likely to have further heart problems.

And let's not forget the preventive aspects of exercise. Studies have shown that people who are physically active have about half the colon cancer risk as those who are sedentary. Evidence also suggests that exercise reduces the risk of breast and prostate cancers by modulating hormone levels.

I'm too old. Forget it. I'm not buying that one. The evidence is very clear that older adults who exercise feel better, live longer, and have fewer physical problems. Even nursing home patients who, by definition, are the frailest of the frail can have threefold improvement in strength when they lift weights. Balance improves and they're much less likely to fall and be injured. Nearly every measure of health improves with exercise.

The ability to exercise does decline with age, of course. You won't be as strong at 70 as you were at 20, and you won't have quite as much endurance. That doesn't matter at all. As long as you're always pushing yourself a little harder and farther, you're going to benefit.

I'm in too much pain. While you don't want to exercise right after an injury, chronic pain, such as that caused by arthritis, is actually improved with exercise. Your pain may affect the kind of exercises you do, but not your ability. Studies have clearly shown that a cornerstone of therapy for back pain involves physical activity, supervised exercise, and stretching. The same is true of arthritis. Believe it or not, more exercise means less pain.

I'm too fat and I look lousy in tights. I can't say I blame anyone who's reluctant to exercise in a gym surrounded by buff 25-year-olds! I have felt this way myself. But look: you cannot let some young dude who spends hours looking at his abs keep you from getting to the gym. If you want to avoid the intimidation-factor, don't go to a Power House gym! Find a local gym that caters to an older clientele. I promise they're out there.

One of my friends, a 25-year-old woman, once told me, "The three older women who work out together at my gym amaze me. They're well into their sixties and they're there more often that I am. I'm not thinking about how they have more wrinkles than me. I'm thinking, my gosh, I want to be that dedicated and active when I'm that age."

I hate to exercise. I hate to say it, but this one's hard to argue with. Some people don't like doing crossword puzzles, some don't like bowling, and others, I'm afraid, don't like to exercise. All I can say is, "Get over it!" You might not like exercise, but I guarantee you'll like having a heart attack a lot less.

When people say they hate to exercise, they usually mean they hate some of specific activity that they associate with "getting into shape." Me, I disliked jogging with a passion. It took me awhile to discover how much I like riding a stationary bike. You'll surely find an exercise that's right for you. It could be biking, swimming, tennis, or walking the dog. If you make the commitment that you're going to exercise *no matter what,* you'll eventually find something that agrees with you.

Creating an exercise program for you

All forms of exercise are beneficial, so it doesn't matter what kind of activity you do. Ultimately, your exercise regimen needs to accomplish two things: increased cardiovascular strength and increased physical strength.

The aerobic edge

Let's start with aerobic exercise, which is any activity that increases your heart and respiratory rates. Aerobic exercise works the most important muscle in your body ... the heart. If you are interested in living a long, healthy life, your heart needs to be as strong as possible. This is only accomplished through aerobic or cardiovascular training.

The American College of Sports Medicine (ACSM) defines aerobic exercise as "any activity that uses large muscle groups, can be maintained continuously, and is rhythmic in nature." For real health and fitness gains, aerobic exercise has to give the heart and lungs a tough workout.

During an aerobic workout, your body responds to maximize the amount of oxygen in your blood. You breathe deeper and faster. Your heart will beat faster and stronger, which maximizes blood flow to your muscles and back to your lungs. Small blood vessels widen to deliver more oxygen to your muscles and carry away waste products, such as carbon dioxide and lactic acid. Your body even releases endorphins, natural painkillers that promote an increased sense of well-being. When you're aerobically fit, your body more efficiently takes in and uses oxygen to sustain movement.

Regular aerobic exercise works the heart just like lunges work your legs. After a while, your heart—like your legs—gets stronger. Think about it like this: Imagine you have 100 pounds of paper that you need to move from one place to the next. The first time you do it, it may take you 20 trips back and forth because you're only strong enough to carry five pounds at a time. But the second time you do it, it only takes you 18 trips. By the tenth time you do it, you can move all hundred pounds of water in five trips – carrying twenty pounds at a time! This is the same way your heart works when you exercise regularly. It may take an unfit heart three or four times the amount of energy to move the same amount of blood as fit heart. A well-exercised heart can pump more blood with less exertion.

Your heart, like your joints, will experience changes as you age. Over time, we will all develop some degree of cholesterol deposi-tions. Even without symptoms, the blockages can be quite exten-sive and it only gets worse with age. A stronger heart can pump more blood through a smaller or blocked vessel. Additionally, reg-ular aerobic exercise increases your good HDL cholesterol while decreasing your bad LDL cholesterol.

In the end, regular aerobic exercise helps prevent heart at-tacks, improves heart function, and reduces the risk of high blood pressure – all of which help you live longer.

In addition to strengthening your heart, aerobic exercise is excellent exercise for the lungs. It helps remove mucus from the airways and can even minimize damage caused by smoking or air pollution.

Perhaps one of the greatest consequences of aerobic exercise is its powerful effect on mood. During cardiovascular training, your body releases endorphins that can improve mood, reduce the risk of depression, and increase energy and work performance. By any objective (and subjective) measure, it improves the quality of life.

Whether you're swimming, jogging, biking, dancing, or walk-ing, the ideal goal is to elevate your heart rate to between 60 and 80% of its top rate. Don't get thrown by the numbers. This is an easy calculation to make. First, subtract your age from 220. If you're 55 years old, for example, your maximum heart rate is somewhere around 165 beats a minute. A good aerobic workout will raise your heart rate to 60 to 80% of that. In this case, that's between 99 and 132 beats a minutes. Plan on maintaining that heart rate for at least 30 minutes, and do it at least three to five days a week.

The most important part of aerobic exercise is choosing something you enjoy. Jogging, swimming, walking, treadmills, and exercise bikes are all good choices, but not necessarily for you. Find what works *for you* and you'll be well on your way to becoming a lifelong exerciser.

Resistance training
People tend to think of weight lifting as a hobby for the young and fit, but it's so much more than that. I can't think of a single lifestyle change that's more beneficial than lifting weights a few times a week.

Weight lifting can dramatically increase muscle size and strength in people of all ages. The benefits of weight training only increase as we get older. New research has shown that nursing home residents who participated in a weight-training program were able to triple their muscle size and strength, while at the same time dramatically reducing risk of falls and fractures. Strength training builds bone *and* muscle—the two things that your body is likely to lose with age.

Whenever I go to the gym, I invariably see a lot of people, young and old, who tend to lift weights that don't appear very challenging. I hate to say it, but just lifting a small dumbbell, one that hardly taxes your reserves, isn't worth the effort. Every study that has shown substantial benefits from resistance training involved high-intensity, muscle-taxing exercises.

In practical terms, this means choosing weights sufficiently heavy for the muscle to be virtually exhausted after six to eight repetitions of the exercise. According to exercise physiologists, you'll get the most benefits when the muscles are "exercised to 80% of a single maximum repetition." Suppose that you choose a weight that's so heavy that you can only lift it once. Obviously, that's too heavy to get much of a workout. You want to start out by lifting 80% of that amount, and repeating the exercise six to eight times.

When you can complete the exercise eight times without being totally exhausted, it's time to increase the weight.

Sound like hard work? It is, believe me. But it's the only way to build your strength to the level it needs for optimal fitness. You'll probably be a little sore when you first start out. But the soreness goes away and you'll soon find that you feel refreshed and energized after your workouts. Your muscles will be tired, but they won't hurt.

Weight training should be done under the supervision of a trainer or physical therapist, at least until you learn the ropes. Unlike walking or biking, which are almost impossible to do wrong, weight training requires proper form and technique. Barbells, dumbbells, and other kinds of free weights provide a superb workout, but they do require more balance, more strength, and more technique than machine weights. If you're adverse to using weights, try elastic bands, which come in varying levels of resistance.

I don't recommend the use of home equipment. Apart from the initial expense, it's hard to stay motivated when your workout room is a musty corner of the basement. Health clubs are a much better choice. There are people on staff who can explain how to use the weights properly and reduce the risk of getting hurt. Health clubs are also a lot of fun because it's a way to get out of the house and meet new people. Don't worry, you won't be the only beginner, and you certainly won't be the only adult over age 30. Those perfect (and intimidating) bodies are the exception, not the rule. Whether you've been active all your life or are just starting out, you and your physique will feel right at home.

Nine steps to more movement

Now that you're sufficiently inspired to start your own exercise program, here are nine steps to get your going.

1. See your doctor first. If haven't exercised much before, or if you're over the age of 65, see your doctor before lacing up the athletic shoes. You want to be sure that you aren't at risk for a sudden heart attack or other health problems when you put your body under more strain than it's accustomed to. If you're really out of shape, you might need to overcome the effects of de-conditioning, a fancy way of saying that you have so little muscle and stamina that even mild exercise leaves you exhausted, breathless, and weak. You may need to work with a physical therapist who will put you on a program of graded exercise, in which you very gradually build up your endurance.

2. Make exercise a priority. Regular exercise is one of the only ways to ensure lifelong health, so make it a priority. You always can make time for what's important—whether that's visiting your kids, calling your mother, or taping *Desperate Housewives*. If your health is important to you, you can always make time for exercise. If it helps, think of your exercise time as *your time*: the time you dedicate to yourself every week to be a little healthier. If you think about all the hours you devote to other people in your life, taking a few hours a week for yourself is not too much to ask.

3. Recruit a friend. Find a friend to get you going. Undertaking any major lifestyle change in pairs is uniformly more successful than going it alone. If you've been sedentary for many years, you're in for a few difficult weeks when you first start exercising. Your body won't be used to moving, and it's going to let you know. I promise you, your mind will rebel. Until exercise becomes a habit, you're going to have to depend on willpower to make it happen. If you have someone else doing it with you, it's a lot easier to stick with the plan and motivate each other. But remember: choose someone who is enthusiastic, motivated, and *reliable*. It's no good working out with someone who is less committed than you or more likely to come up with excuses. Sorry to say it, but the perfect exercise partner may not be your best friend.

4. Create a realistic schedule. Remember, fitness does not have to be an all-or-nothing pursuit. Don't jump out there planning to work out six days a week. Over-committing is a recipe for failure. Once you start missing your exercise sessions, you inevitable feel guilty and like you failed. Keep your schedule simple and one you can stick to.

5. Hire a trainer or coach. Every skill worth mastering—whether it's playing an instrument or learning to meditate—requires outside help and guidance. Exercise is no exception. Hire a well-qualified fitness trainer to help you get started. He or she will keep you motivated and ensure you maintain proper form. Tell your trainer you want to combine aerobic exercise with resistance training. Too often we avoid lifting weights, which is a major no-no for the aging body. When you go looking for a fitness trainer, ask about her credentials and see if she has worked with someone your age. Trust me, you do not want a trainer who treats your body like it's 25! Not only is that irresponsible, it's dangerous and you could hurt yourself.

6. Do something you enjoy! There are many different ways to exercise, so it's absolutely imperative that you find something you enjoy. Fitness should be challenging, but not miserable or painful. Remember that your body may not be suited for every fitness pursuit. What's more, you may need to alter your work-outs as you age. Running may have been great at 25, but it could really be painful at 50. Whatever you do, find an activity that suits your body; that's the only way you'll really enjoy it. For me the best exercise is walking and biking, but if you have joint pains you may want to consider swimming. You can exercise outside or at a gym—it doesn't matter. Do what works for you and stick with it.

7. Start slow but keep at it. Even though 30 minutes or more of aerobic exercise is ideal, you should think of this as a target to aim for, rather than something to achieve immediately. If you've been sedentary for a long time, plan on doing some brisk aerobic exercise for 10 to 15 minutes. If you're breathless, you're pushing too hard and need to back off. Don't get discouraged. Use the "talking test" as a measure of how hard you're working: if you can talk easily and keep up a conversation, you're not working hard enough. If you're huffing and puffing and out of breath, you're working too hard. You should be able to talk, but you should be working hard enough that you just don't want to! Listen to your body and do not over-exert yourself out of the gates.

Your ultimate goal should be to aerobically exercise three to four days a week and resistance train at least twice. Remember that you can combine cardio and strength training into one longer workout. Ideally, your aerobic exercise should last at least 30 minutes a day and you're your weight training should work your muscles to exhaustion. When lifting weights, aim for three sets of 10 repetitions each. If the 10th repetition is not very difficult, the weight is too low. Once again, always use proper form to avoid injury. Muscle soreness is okay … pain is not. If something hurts, stop doing it and look for another exercise.

8. Set goals and aim high. Begin with a few baby steps, but set your expectations high. Each and every one of us has our own mountain to climb. For some, the peak is as high as the Himalayas. For others, it's the height of a curb. As long as you take those first steps, you'll see amazing progress. Set specific short-term and long-term goals and share them with a friend, a relative, or your trainer.

9. Reward yourself! Once you've achieved a goal—whether it's the goal for the day, the week, or the year—reward yourself. Fitness should be fun and enjoyable! Don't get so caught up in someone else's definition of what it means to be fit; you're climbing your very own, unique mountain. Once you get there, enjoy the view!

CHAPTER 10
BE MORE EMPOWERED ABOUT YOUR HEALTH

We live in an age of overwhelming consumerism, from cars to houses, mutual funds to education. Americans today have a veritable avalanche of options! And, for the most part, we exercise the right to shop around. We search exhaustively for the best deal, research every decision, and weigh every option. Industries respond with more disclosure and more refined competition. In the end, the American consumer is a savvy shopper, a force to be reckoned with! That is … until he or she steps into the doctor's office.

Once you see that white coat and the M.D at the end of your doctor's name, all bets are off! The comparison ends, the savvy demands diminish, and you place all your faith in this "highly trained" and "supremely confident" physician. It's crazy! Doctors are fallible human beings; many of them have loads of patients and stressful lives. Mistakes can happen and, sadly, not everyone follows the same standard practices of care. *You* are responsible for your own healthcare! When it comes to taking control of your health, you cannot focus on lifestyle issues alone. At some point, you must engage with the traditional medical system and be empowered about your care *and* your options. For baby boomers who are classically described as the "most educated, most affluent, and most demanding" generation, we must not abandon that mentality after entering our doctor's office.

For each decade after 50 years of age, being empowered about your health becomes more and more important. As we age, the risk of developing a chronic illness progressively rises. But remember that your age does not determine your quality of life. It is your health that holds the key to longevity and independence. Illness is the culprit in "age-related" issues. Whether it be high blood pressure, heart disease, stroke, cancer, kidney failure, arthritis or back pain, these *conditions* make you feel "old." Disease makes us dependent, disease forces us into hospitals or nursing homes, and disease shortens our lives.

Clearly (and quite obviously), the key to living a healthy and happy life is to be disease-free! My goal, as both a geriatrician and a patient, is to accomplish two tasks:

1. Prevent disease from occurring at all
2. Make sure I identify and treat any illness as early as possible.

The only way to accomplish this goal is to become a truly empowered and impassioned consumer of health care. Throughout this book, I'm emphasizing every possible way that *you* can prevent disease, by living a healthy life, by eating right, by exercising, and by being passionate about each day. But sooner or later, all of us must come in to contact with the health care system. Regardless of the personal lifestyle changes, there will be times that you must turn yourself over to a physician for help, guidance, and therapy. What then? Do you throw away your own sense of choice or power? *No!* In any relationship, including the one with your physician, you must remain impassioned and empowered about your own health.

The ninth step in Dr. David's Longevity plan is to be *more* empowered! In the following pages, I outline the major problems with American health care along with clear tips to help you navigate the system. You will also find a detailed description of what to expect of your doctor. Use this as your basic checklist to get started.

Ultimately, there are two main steps to being an empowered consumer of health care:

1. Understand the pitfalls of American health care
2. Learn to navigate the system

First, you must understand what you're up against …

The envy of the world? What's wrong with the American health care system?

In 2004, President George W. Bush stated, "The US health care system is the envy of the world." But how envious should the world be, really? Consider this: America spends five times more on health care than any other developed country in the world, yet we rank 29th in the overall health of our citizens, nearly *last* among all developed countries. Despite all the money we spend on curing disease, we rank 42nd in longevity! Dig a little deeper in to the data and you will find that longevity is not just an "American" issue, but a socioeconomic and ethnic one as well. The life expectancy among affluent whites (77.9 years of age) competes well with most countries in Asia and Europe. However, the average life expectancy of black males averages 69 years, lower than Cuba, Iran, and Syria.

Perhaps the most alarming statistic of all is that the United States has a higher rate of infant mortality than most other developed countries. We rank 41st behind most developed Asian countries, Europe and Cuba.

The medical-industrial complex
In his farewell speech to the nation, President Eisenhower warned Americans against "the military-industrial complex" and "the potential for the disastrous rise of misplaced power." At the time, his words were a shockingly direct challenge to system, and a concept that flew in face of traditional power. He was right ... and Americans took note.

But over forty years later, a new threat has eclipsed that of even the military-industrial complex. Today, it is the **medical-industrial complex** of which Americans should be wary. The close relationship between health care, private industry, and political or commercial interest has exerted enormous influence on they way we practice medicine. In my view, it has hindered everyone from receiving rational, affordable, and accessible care.

The biggest problem with the medical-industrial complex is that it created a market-based approach to medicine where the bottom line is paramount. The impact of this shift can be seen in every facet of care, from physicians and patients to policymakers and insurers. From the purely medical point of view, American health care centers on high-technology, acute care medicine. We focus on cutting-edge treatments and procedures that fuel the big business of health care, but add to skyrocketing costs for consumers. The insurance industry follows suit by rewarding physicians for using these expensive procedures and pays very little (or nothing at all) for the routine and necessary services of disease detection and prevention. As a result, everyone neglects the less sexy, less profitable business of prevention and primary medicine. Medical students run from family practice and geriatrics, choosing rather to pursue the high-dollar business of sub-specialty care such as cardiology and orthopedics.

From a consumer perspective, individuals want the "best" and the newest treatments, especially because insurance pays for it. Thanks to savvy marketing campaigns, patients often request the newest and most expensive technologies and medications, allowing physicians to charge more money and try a new therapy, even without sufficient evidence to support its value.

In turn, this is great for big pharmaceutical and other health-care companies, which justify the large price tag by huge research budgets required to identify a new treatment and bring it to the marketplace. American politicians and policymakers see this as the very best of "free-market medicine," and choose not to regulate the price of therapy. Unfortunately, because every other developed country imposes strong regulations and limits the price an individual will pay for a new therapy, this forces Americans to shoulder a disproportionate share of the bulky research budgets.

In the end, medicine has become susceptible to the laws of supply and demand. The medical-industrial complex has created a vicious cycle where we all carry some responsibility for the problems in American health care. While politicians must combat these problems on a policy level and physicians must combat them from a medical perspective, *you* must combat them by being educated and empowered about your health. If you blindly trust your physician and buy in to the hype of "modern medicine" or high-technology care, your health could be compromised.

Beyond the rhetoric: the REAL consequences of being less empowered

Beyond the rhetoric, there are real consequences of being a disempowered consumer of health care. The cycle of the medical-industrial complex relies on an uneducated patient. It will not work if you demand a rational and affordable approach to treatment. Just think about it: the health care system is confusing, elitist, and often extremely frustrating. It is not exactly conducive to an individual taking charge, so patients must put all of their trust in a physician who may or may not be acting in their best interests. To make matters worse, once you face a major illness, it is very difficult to ask your doctor the reason for anything being done, especially when he or she says that this test or this procedure will save your life.

Although I see patients struggle to navigate the health system every day, the following story really shook me. It is a classic example of the medical-industrial complex at work. In my mind, this family endured the very worst of American health care. It further confirms my belief that being an empowered consumer of health care should be required reading before ever stepping foot in a doctor's office.

In 2006, I wrote a column about HeartSaver CT screenings. These screening tests identify calcium deposits in coronary arteries shown to be a good predictor of increased risk of coronary artery disease. The idea is that you can avoid a major heart attack through early detection and therapy. While this machine certainly has great potential to detect disease and prevent illness, it also comes with a degree of risk. Once you know that you have a problem, it opens the door for physicians to recommend invasive therapy, which may not be necessary. And nothing scares a patient more than heart disease! So of course you are going to support any decision you physician recommends. To make this issue even more complicated, many of the HeartSaver CT machines are owned by cardiologists. So physicians may be more inclined to promote the more expensive and profitable surgery, rather than prescribe lifestyle changes and medication. The bottom line of the article was to alert patients that there are a variety of options available. Depending on your age, symptoms, and family history, you should not immediately assume surgery is the best path. Later in this chapter, I'll talk more about the dangers of invasive therapy for heart disease, but first read this letter I received accounting one daughter's devastating run-in with the HeartSaver CT and an aggressive cardiologist.

These are her words:

> *I just read your article in Sunday's Arkansas Democrat Gazette. I feel certain the person you are talking about is my mother. She and I went the day before Thanksgiving to the heart hospital and had a "heart saver" test. After the CAT scan was done we were told she had lots of calcium in her coronary artery. She then had an appointment with a cardiologist who ran tests and said she needed bypass surgery immediately. He sent her to a surgeon, who did surgery a week later on 12-6-05.*
>
> *She stayed in the hospital until 12-11-05 after having quadruple bypass surgery. When she finally came home, she never felt good, her heart pounded the whole time, so we returned to the emergency room on 12-16-05 and she had emergency surgery that night. She had a blood clot behind her aorta. She then suffered a major stroke and is now paralyzed on her right side, cannot speak, has a catheter and a feeding tube.*
>
> *She was never given any option other than surgery. Before this, she was a very energetic lady who loved life and was continually doing things at church, home, etc. She is 77 years old. My sister and I were heartsick after reading your article. If only we had known BEFORE her surgery. If only we had known there were alternatives, she would have her health now. It is so sad especially to know it could have been prevented. My sister's husband had people come up to him today and ask if this article was about his mother-in-law. Hopefully, people will stop and think before they have unnecessary surgery. We did talk to another patient's family while at the hospital who told us the same story. We (my sister and I) have so many unanswered questions. Thanks for informing people. Hopefully, they will listen and not end up like us.*
>
> *Sincerely,*
> *Phyllis Cash*

Since receiving the letter, I have kept in close touch with Phyllis. Her mother resided in a nursing home until she finally died in July 2007. During her nursing home stay, her husband completely depleted his nest egg to support the high price of private care. Today, he no longer lives on his own and struggles to make ends meet.

I am so saddened by this family's story. Mrs. Cash's mother—vibrant and asymptomatic when first screened—did not need any of the invasive surgeries that ultimately left her paralyzed, bedbound, and in need of fulltime care. When the doctor said, "You need immediate surgery to save your life," of course she and her children felt they had no options but surgery.

As far as I'm concerned, the Cashes are victims of the medical-industrial complex. The HeartSaver CT screening was new and exciting, a great breakthrough in medicine! And yet for a woman like Mrs. Cash it was not considered a necessary or *recommended* screening. Despite this, thousands of people flocked to take advantage of this cutting-edge therapy and many of them ended up in the operating room without ever attempting to address less-invasive methods of treating heart disease. The United States Preventative Task Force maintains that there is no place for the HeartSaver CT scan in the screening for coronary artery disease. One could make a case for the value of identifying calcium in coronary arteries in high-risk individuals in their 40s, 50s, and early 60s, but screening someone over the age of 70 is flat wrong. Autopsy studies indicate that more than 50% of the population will have coronary artery disease and there is no evidence to indicate that surgery offers any benefit for asymptomatic older adults in preventing heart attacks or prolonging life. In fact, the risk of complications after surgery is much higher than the risk of succumbing to a heart attack. Mrs. Cash failed to get a second opinion or consult her primary physician; rather she chose to put all her trust in an aggressive cardiologist and the value of cutting-edge medicine.

This is the problem with American Healthcare. As we age, it is only going to get worse.

If you simply roll all responsibility over to your doctor, chances are you will have too many expensive tests, which will be performed far too frequently, and you may be monitored by unneeded scans that inundate you with an unhealthy amount of radiation. Five Heartsaver CT scans provide as much irradiation as if you were 60 miles away from ground zero when the bomb exploded in Hiroshima! Your physician may recommend unnecessary surgeries or interventions. In many instances, you will not be given options, nor will you be informed about expected benefits and potential side effects. Regardless, you can rest assured that your physician will prescribe the newest, most expensive drug over the generic, tried-and-true options.

Medicine is no longer the noble profession

Dr. Thomas E. Andreoli, a giant in the field of medicine, died recently. He will be sorely missed. His obituary described him as unashamedly "old school" where honor, integrity, service, the needs of the patient and scholarship were the highest priority. Those were the days. Physicians were well paid but mercantile issues were never a serious consideration and wide disparities in the value of the primary care doctor whose knowledge and insight were critical to patient care was not that different from the subspecialist, surgeon or radiologist who performed sophisticated procedures to diagnose, treat and yes cure disease.

How things have changed! Today medicine is a business and the bottom line has become ever more important. The most successful physicians are the entrepreneurs who understand how to run their practices with a major focus on profit. These days physicians band together as subspecialty and multispecialty groups and have put in place a model where profit is generated not only from the fees paid by commercial insurance companies and Medicare for the hands-on patient care, but also from the array of tests that are so readily ordered on every patient. These groups own their own equipment and facilities and make a profit by ordering blood tests, imaging studies such as CT scans and MRIs, and—based upon the results (for which pay is quite handsome)—more invasive procedures and expensive therapies are recommended.

Here is an example: an 82-year-old woman went for an annual physical by her internist who is a member of a large multispecialty group. She had a five-minute visit with a nurse in which a few questions were asked and a series of laboratory tests were ordered (as was an EKG, a stress test and an echocardiogram). The patient did have some heart problems and these tests were performed annually. Three weeks later, a 10-minute follow-up visit reassured her she was doing well. The cost and reimbursement to the doctor were substantial. Most tests were unnecessary. Another example is an 81-year-old man with severe lung disease receiving oxygen at rest. Although about to enter a hospice program, he had recently seen a urologist for an elevated PSA suggesting prostate cancer. Amazingly, a biopsy of his prostate was planned in the next few weeks.

I could fill a book with examples of care that I and most other rational physicians would view as unnecessary. In the old-school days, these practices were virtually never seen. Not surprisingly, health care providers are losing the public's trust as everyone recognizes that something is truly unhealthy about our broken health care system. We accept that doctors do too much but feel powerless to do anything when "too much" is done to us. How are we to know or question the wisdom of the physician who suggests an approach to care that may or may not be in our best interests?

The loss of trust in health care providers may have disastrous effects in the future. Physicians are playing a very small role in health care reform. And their role is largely to protect the bottom line by assuring payment for latest most expensive care that must be available to everyone. As payment for individual health care services are cut back, the impetus for physicians to do more unnecessary care to meet the bottom line will only increase. In the end the system will fail and health care may emerge in a drastically different form with few opportunities for innovation, new discoveries and cures.

I urge physicians to think about how good things were in the old-school days. We must regain public trust by being responsible, honorable, and ethical, and assure that we do the right thing. Work toward only practicing medicine that is truly necessary, educate our patients and be accountable for containing costs. In the old-school days, a leader like Tom Andreoli would identify the solution and never abrogate that responsibility to politicians, public policy experts and others who have no hands-on patient care experience. It will take leaders like him to ensure that medicine remains the noble profession, meeting the needs of the population without breaking the bank.

As a consumer of health care, you must recognize the sorry state of the system. Reading this, you may think, "I'd better just stay away!" But despite all these problems, avoiding the health system altogether is a very dangerous decision.

Remember, I tell everyone over the age of 50 the same thing: "The healthier you are today, the more you need me." You do not want to wait until illness strikes to engage with the health care system. If you are healthy today, take the time *now* to develop a trusting relationship with a good primary physician.

Now that you understand the challenges of the American medicine, you can develop the tools to navigate the system and empower *yourself* to be healthy.

Navigating the health system

Have you ever heard the saying, "Your body is like a fine sports car. The more you take care of it, the better it will perform"? Well, it is true. As your body becomes "vintage," you need those regular check-ups to make sure everything is in order. Just like a classic car, as we age, complications become more likely. And if you wait until the engine falls out, it may be too late!

Whenever you ultimately choose to engage with the traditional medical system, you must be empowered from the get-go. Before you even enter the doctor's office, consider these tips:

- **Don't believe everything your doctor tells you.** Too many of us blindly place our doctor on a pedestal. Remember, you are a paying customer. But unlike your lawyer or your accountant, your doctor is not paid by the time spent with you. Pay is based on the complexity of the visit. Ask questions, demand answers, and seek second opinions whenever necessary. Remember that physicians are fallible, have biases, and if they have the expertise to order or perform expensive procedures, they will definitely be more liberal in recommending them. It's just human nature.

- **Be wary of tests.** Ask your physician why you need a test, what he or she hopes to find, and what data exists to support this course of action. Many screening tests are routinely prescribed even though scientific evidence fails to support their value. It is imperative that you know what tests are appropriate, how often you should have them, and why. The more tests your doctor orders, particularly if he does them in his office or uses machines he owns the more he gets paid.

- **Be educated about your illness.** The key to being an educated and empowered consumer of health care is taking it upon yourself to research and understand any illness. If you are internet-savvy, get online and scour the web for reliable information. Only use websites, however, that are supported by reputable institutions such as the Mayo Clinic, WebMD, Medscape, etc. Demand that your physician adequately explain every element of your condition, including the desired therapy, medications, and course of action. Then go back to your research and compare your physician's prescribed therapy to the recommended guidelines set forth by any major national health group, such as the American Heart Association.

Engage early

For baby boomers, to begin the process of navigating the health system, you must first ***engage early***. This simply means that you cannot wait until disaster strikes to develop a good relationship with a physician. By engaging early, you can be vigilant about the little things and prevent the major problems from ever arising. So if you truly seek to be passionate about your health, I strongly recommend you launch a thorough search for a knowledgeable, qualified, and humble physician.

You need to know the who, what, when, where, and why of your medical check-up. *When* should you go to the doctor? *Who* should you see and *where* should you go? *What* should you expect and *why*?

In order to engage early, I suggest you begin with an annual physical. This will accomplish two tasks: 1) you can determine exactly how healthy you really are, and 2) you can assess your physician and determine if it's a good long-term fit.

An annual physical or routine medical check up can vary wildly, from cursory exams to intensive total body screenings. So I am going to demystify the doctor's office, pull back the curtains, and give you a step-by-step account of a quality medical exam.

When should you go to the doctor?

As a general rule, you should be thoroughly evaluated at the age of 50 and probably every two or three years until age 65. After 65, you should have an annual medical check-up. If you develop a medical problem of some relevance, such as high blood pressure, severe arthritis, or a chronic condition such as fibromyalgia, more frequent visits to the doctor may be needed.

If you are approaching your 65th birthday, Medicare provides a onetime benefit that allows a comprehensive history and physical examination as well as an extended list of screenings to identify commonly occurring medical conditions. However, there is fine print with Medicare's once-in-a-lifetime offer: you must take advantage of this benefit within 6 months of your 65th birthday.

For individuals at high risk of illness, you may consider having an annual exam as early at 30 years of age. If you have any of these risk factors, you should seriously consider close and persistent monitoring by your trusted physician:

- **Family history of heart disease, stroke, high blood pressure, diabetes, or cancer.** This is especially serious if any conditions presented at an early age. If your father had a heart attack at age 40, you fall into this category. Breast, colon, prostate cancer, or melanoma can be hereditary. The rarer cancers such as those occurring in the brain or kidney, leukemias, and lymph-node cancers are less likely to occur in families. The more family members who present with problems under the age of 60, the more important that you are closely monitored.

- **High blood pressure.** Go to the supermarket and take your blood pressure. If the top (systolic) value is above 135 or the bottom (diastolic) is above 90, you should consider seeing a doctor.

- **High cholesterol.** At some point before the age of 30, you should have your cholesterol checked. If the total is above 200 and the bad (LDL) cholesterol is above 130, you should consider seeing a physician. There is compelling evidence that the earlier high cholesterol levels are identified and corrected, the greater the reduction in risk of heart attack and stroke.

- **Being overweight.** If you are 50 pounds overweight or have a BMI of greater than 30, you should see a physician for a complete history and physical. Being seriously overweight is usually a step toward other serious diseases. (Remember, there is no such thing as a weight problem—just a health problem!)

- **Smoking.** If you are smoker, be seen by a physician frequently. While there really is no test to detect lung cancer early, smokers are at much greater risk of heart disease, stroke, and a number of common cancers, including bladder, colon and prostate.

- **Using drugs or alcohol.** If you have a problem with drugs and alcohol or have been told you drink too much, seek medical help. Many illnesses can be caused or aggravated by alcohol or other drug use.

No matter your age, never ignore a new symptom. If you are concerned about a problem, never sweep it under the rug, because it may be serious. Any form of chest pain may be a harbinger of heart disease, a bad headache may be dangerous, and many other warning signs of illness can lead to early detection of disease.

Who should you see and where should you go?
If you are over the age of 65, consider a senior health center.
Many hospitals today are developing senior health centers with hospital-employed physicians. Senior health centers typically are staffed with geriatricians who fully understand the unique needs of an aging adult. In addition, these centers generally employ a team-based approach to care, keeping pharmacists, social workers, dieticians, and other health-care professionals on staff. In addition, because their income is not dependent on the pure number of patients seen, salaried physicians often feel less pressure to order tests or conduct extra procedures. Most importantly, these doctors typically can spend more time per patient and place a large emphasis on early detection and prevention. At the Donald W. Reynolds Senior Health Center, each new patient is allocated *a full hour* for an initial consult, and thirty minutes for follow-ups.

To be honest, senior health centers are not opened for purely altruistic reasons, because hospitals have a vested interest in providing quality care to older adults. Research conducted at the Donald W. Reynolds Department of Geriatrics shows that hospitals with robust senior health centers see a huge benefit in downstream revenue. Adults over the age of 65 are the greatest users of health care, so our patients inevitably utilize services elsewhere in the hospital system. Therefore, our goal is not to see as many patients as possible, but rather to create a long-lasting, trusting relationship with every patient.

If you are under the age of 65, diligently seek out a physician who is willing to give you time and attention. Find someone who respects your questions and input. If your physician balks at the suggestion of a second opinion, find a new doctor. Any physician should encourage and empower you to seek additional information and advice. If they don't, something may be wrong.

What should you expect and why?
The intensity of the annual examination can vary a great deal. A screening done at a major hospital like the Mayo Clinic may involve evaluations by multiple physicians, having a large number of blood tests, x-rays, imaging studies (such as CT scans), EKG, echocardiogram and a treadmill stress test. At the other extreme, some annual physicals offer a perfunctory examination with very little done at all. Because of the fast-paced, bottom-line-driven business of health care, many patients are shortchanged when they see their doctor for an initial visit. You will often spend more time with office staff than with your physician and get little opportunity to discuss your health, history, and concerns.

Rather than being passive and trusting your physician to do whatever he or she deems best, you can take steps to be well prepared before ever putting on the paper gown. Know what tests to expect, what questions to be asked, and how much you can expect to pay.

Every patient should take this simple first step: **Tell your physician that you seek to be truly educated about how to stay healthy and reduce your risk of illness.** This is important because it will let your doctor know that you are serious about prevention and willing to take every possible step to avoid illness.

Here's a tip: if you are over the age of 50 and your first visit does not entail at least 40 minutes of face time with your physician, it is not likely thorough enough and potential problems could be missed. Before coming to any diagnoses or determining if additional tests are needed, your physician must take a comprehensive history and perform a thorough head to toe examination.

THE HISTORY

- **Main complaints.** Is anything bothering you and, if so, what symptoms do you complain of? Each of your concerns should be discussed in detail. Questions asked will depend on the problem. Each response could lead to a unique diagnosis. A good doctor will be thorough, not rush, and spend as much time discussing each complaint as needed. By the end, you should feel like your complaints were heard, validated, and understood.

- **Medications.** Your doctor must go over each and every medication you take, whether they are prescribed, over the counter, an alternative therapy (such as ginko biloba or any other "natural product") or a nutritional supplement including vitamins and minerals. Simply looking at the medications a patient takes immediately identifies any past or present medical problems. Your doctor should understand how your various medications may be interacting.

- **Past medical history.** Your physician should document all the surgeries you have had as well as every admission to a hospital during your lifetime.

- **Family history.** Your doctor should ask for a comprehensive family health history. Including asking if your parents are still alive and, if not, why they died and how old they were at their time of death. Any problems in your siblings, children and other close relatives should be recorded, as should a family history of heart disease, high blood pressure, cancer, diabetes and Alzheimer's disease – all of which are more common in family members.

- **Social history.** Your doctor should know as much about you as possible. Are you married and for how long? Did you attend college? What work do you do? Are you happy and do you have any hobbies? Are you sexually active and are there any problems? Is religion important in your life? Understanding all of these elements allows a good physician to understand your comprehensive state of health.

- **Habits.** Understanding your lifestyle habits is an important component of assessing your health risks. Do you smoke, how many cigarettes daily, and for how long? Do you drink alcohol, how many glasses a day, and has it ever been a problem?

- **Review of systems.** Your physician should delve into any symptoms that may relate to a particular organ system. This will help determine if you have any problems with your overall health and provide clues if a problem exists involving an organ system such as the heart, lung, gastrointestinal system, neurological system, or bones, muscles and joints.

THE EXAMINATION
The first time you see your doctor, he or she should examine you in great detail from head to toe. The more thorough, the better. Through this detailed and compulsive process, your physician may recognize problems that you did not discuss earlier. For example, I often have identified narrowing of the carotid artery and noted heart murmurs that the patient never knew existed. A detailed

description of critical aspects of the examination is shown in the Section B of the appendix.

SCREENING TESTS

Based upon the information obtained during your examination and history, your doctor should know almost as much about you as after blood tests and other screening tests are done. Your risk factor of illness will determine how aggressively you will be screened for diseases. Screening tests are an important component of nearly every medical check-up; it is imperative, however, that your physician educate you about why each test is done, what should you expect, and what evidence exists to support that course of action.

Section A in the appendix details the current guidelines for screening tests recommended by the United States Preventative Services Task Force. I'll talk more about screening tests later in this chapter

ASSESSMENT AND PLAN

The more information your doctor has, the more likely he or she will identify all of your problems and be able to appropriately counsel you on developing a successful health plan. Before leaving the doctor's office, you should know what you need to do to treat any identified problems, what tests are needed to exclude other medical decisions, and what lifestyle changes are necessary to stay healthy and happy. Your doctor should itemize every actual or potential medical problem that you have or are at risk of developing.

In addition, based upon the assessment, your physician should develop a plan to evaluate the severity of the conditions identified and to exclude any other medical concerns that might be unmasked by additional tests.

A good physician will send you a letter that describes his findings and includes the results of all the tests that were ordered as well as any future plans.

FOLLOW-UP VISITS

At the second visit, your doctor should go over all of your tests in detail, explain any identified problems, and discuss the plan for treatment. At this visit, you should be counseled on the non-medical aspects of lifelong health: the importance of controlling stress and being happy, exercising, eating right, and staying involved in your community. Usually, you will not be examined at your second visit.

For any subsequent visits, you should receive another detailed evaluation with an updated review of complaints and any changes your health history.

At a minimum, my examination at *every* visit includes:

- A blood pressure taken sitting and standing

- Assessing your pulse and cardiac rate

- Making sure that you are not anemic or jaundiced

- Examine the carotid artery and make sure there are no enlarged lymph nodes in the neck

- Examine and listen to the lungs

- Examine and listen to the heart

- Feel the abdomen, make sure there are no masses and that the liver and spleen are not enlarged

- Listen for bruits (turbulence) over the aorta

- Feel the pulses in the leg

A follow-up and history can readily be accomplished in about 20 minutes, which is just enough time to be thorough.

A quick glance at screenings

- At age 50 a single EKG should be done

- Stress testing, echocardiograms and CAT scasn of the heart to screen for heart disease are not recommended in asymptomatic healthy individuals.

- Measure your blood pressure twice yearly.

- Screen for an elevated lipid at age 30 and every five years from age 50

- Screening for an abdominal aortic aneurysm is recommended on one occasion at age 65. Particularly for men and for anyone who has been a significant smoker.

- Screening for blocked carotid arteries is not recommended for asymptomatic healthy individuals.

- There is compelling evidence for mammograms and pelvic and pap smears to exclude breast and gynecological malignancy.

- Screening for colorectal cancer involves annual screening for fecal occult blood and a colonoscopy every 10 years unless risk factors for colorectal cancer are increased.

- The value for digital rectal examination and PSA to screen for prostate cancer remains controversial.

- A bone density to screen for osteoporosis should be done on all women at age 50 and every five years thereafter. Because osteoporosis does occur in men screening should be considered at age 60 and every 5 years thereafter. If there are other risk factors for osteoporosis such as steroid use, or illnesses associated with osteoporosis screening should be done more frequently.

- Certain blood tests to screen for anemia, kidney, thyroid disease, and a number of other conditions may be needed at various intervals ranging from annually to every five years.

Facing illness? Stay engaged!

By learning what to expect from your doctor—and empowering yourself to demand affordable, accessible, and rational care—you can truly embrace the entire spectrum of living a healthy life. By engaging with the health system early and using it to detect and prevent disease, you are leaps and bounds ahead of the majority of Americans. What's more, you no longer have to fear the traditional medical system. Now you know how to work it.

But what happens when you face a serious illness or disease? As I said earlier, many people lose all sense of empowerment when dealing with a health crisis. It's all well and good to have a regular physical exam, but sometimes illnesses pop up when you least expect them.

If and when your doctor does identify an illness, it is very important that you be *passionately involved* in every aspect of care. Do not disengage because you're scared! Remember the story of Mrs. Cash's mother, who rushed to the operating room because a doctor told her it was her only chance for survival! Illness of any kind is scary. It puts one off-balance and makes everyone vulnerable. If the face of *any* health condition, from the life-threatening to the seemingly benign, you must be even more vigilant to ensure appropriate medical care. Every decision must be made carefully, with as much knowledge and insight as possible. In any case, I seriously recommend you solicit the help of a family member or close friend to help you through the process. It is often more difficult to ask the hard questions, be persistent, and demand answers under challenging conditions.

When facing illness, you can really put your new knowledge about the medical-industrial complex to the test. **The biggest challenge is to not fall prey to the idea that new is better than old or more is better than less.**

<u>Sometimes it should be "in with the old, out with the new"</u>
When George Bush spoke about the American health system being the envy of the world, he was right in one aspect: we have the newest, coolest, and most innovative therapies available. If you have a

life-threatening, super-rare condition, come to America. I'm sure that some brilliant physician or scientist has come up with a new, cutting-edge therapy. Every day, specialist physicians in America almost literally bring people back from death's door. We have robot-controlled surgery centers and heart pumps that promise to work better than transplants. We have the newest drugs and the best machines.

Whether it's heart disease or cancer, high blood pressure or stroke, chronic renal failure or diabetes, the technologies to diagnose and treat any medical condition are highly sophisticated and allow the examination of remarkable detail. Based on this technology, it is possible to accurately define the severity and extent of almost any medical problem and come up with a treatment plan that is appropriate, rational, and makes sense for you and your family.

Honestly, this *is* wonderful technology. Americans are at the very forefront of medical innovation—and, for that, we should be proud. But this wonderful technology comes with a cost. Newer typically means expensive. It also means untried. Remember, new drugs and medications must go through very rigorous testing to receive FDA approval. This is not true for new equipment or therapy (such as the HeartSaver CT). In addition, with the market-based approach of the American health system, physicians, administrators, pharmacists, and other health professionals are swayed by the bottom line. Remember, health care is a profit-driven industry, just like anything else. So new therapies often mean more profit.

In recent years, we have seen many examples of how newer doesn't necessarily mean better. First, let's look at the impact of using new, patented medications over older, generic varieties. New drugs enter the market after extensive research and approval from the FDA. However, despite the rigor of FDA approval, it often takes years before we truly understand every side effect of a medication. Just think of the Vioxx fiasco. Vioxx was considered a miracle drug in relieving pain without causing inflammation of the stomach (as seen with older non-steroidal anti-inflammatory drugs or NSAIDs). Once it reached the market, nearly every physician was prescribing this drug for all kinds of pain. A few years and 20 million prescriptions later, the manufacturer announced a worldwide recall after a clinical trial uncovered a potentially fatal side effect: Vioxx caused an unacceptable increased risk of heart attacks. One report published on *The Lancet* website and sponsored by the FDA showed that low doses of Vioxx increased risk of heart attach by almost 50%. In the end, the manufacturer, Merck and Co., was found liable for the death of a man who took Vioxx, and was forced to award his widow $253.4 million in damages! What happened next? Physicians went back to the tried-and-true generic drugs of naprosyn and Motrin, which—when used appropriately—work well for relieving pain.

Vioxx is certainly not the only new medication to cause more harm than good. Many physicians consistently choose to prescribe the newer, fancier drug over the older, generic models. More recently, the newer anti-diabetic drug Actos has been shown to cause a high risk of heart attacks and frequently accelerates the development of osteoporosis.

In many instances, the older therapies are cheaper, more predictable, and often have fewer side effects. Though it may not be the best solution for your specific condition, always ask your doctor about generic drugs and do your own research about recommended therapies. Above all, don't fall prey to savvy marketing campaigns that seduce patients into thinking one drug is better than another! Ask a physician you trust … and get a second opinion.

When it comes to therapy, the issue of new versus old affects medical interventions as well. This is no more evident than in the case of drug-coated stents, a promising, multi-billion dollar industry that continues to face serious problems as the technique evolves.

In 2003, Johnson and Johnson released the first form of a drug-coated stent, a tiny metal scaffold used to reopen blocked arteries in patients with heart disease. Unlike the older, metal stents, these new stents are coated with drugs that prevent the damaged artery from gradually blocking again, a process referred to as restenosis.

The drug-coated stent may reduce the risk of restenosis by 50%, lessening the need for further angiograms and open heart surgery. At the time, cardiologists were so thrilled about the new scientific breakthrough that they implanted 50,000 drug-coated stents within the first three months following its approval. Over the next several years, doctors continued to use more and more of these drug-coated devices and on a wider array of patients.

While the new stents seemed more effective than traditional metal stents, they were also more expensive—costing $2,200. With nearly 1.5 million Americans receiving a stent each year, this means big business! Pharmaceutical companies are generating six billion dollars a year in sales and billions more in hospital and professional fees.

In September 2006 the FDA issued a statement indicating that some patients suffered from an increased risk of sudden blockage of the artery containing the drug-coated stent, which caused a heart attack and high risk of death. It has been reported that incidence of complete blockage of the drug coated stent occurs in about one in 500 cases. But this value may be three to four times higher in routine clinical practice. If this is true, drug-coated stents could lead to a minimum of 2100 deaths from heart attacks every year.

In the case of drug-coated stents, there are some important messages. Physicians were a little too eager to accept the great promise of a new therapy. Today, drug-coated stents are used less often and the pharmaceutical industry continues to tweak and improve this therapy. Ultimately, drug-coated stents may be the best intervention available, far eclipsing the efficacy of the traditional metal stent. However, the intervention is still evolving!

When it comes to medical treatments of any kind, we must all embrace a more skeptical attitude toward new, cutting-edge therapy. This is one of the biggest challenges to navigating the health system. As the consumer, you have a responsibility to question when new is necessary. By that same token, your physician also has the responsibility to know when to prescribe the new over the old … or vice-versa.

<u>When less is more</u>
In addition to the problems of assuming new medicine is better than old, perhaps the greatest misconception in American medicine is that *more* is better than *less*. More surgery, more medicine, more therapy is better than watching, waiting, or doing the least amount of medical intervention possible.

This is especially true when dealing with heart disease. See a cardiologist for a symptom suggestive of a heart problem, and you can rest assured that you'll receive nearly every sophisticated test possible. And if anything is found, your physician is more likely to suggest invasive techniques over conservative therapy. In America, over one million angioplasties are conducted every year.

With all the advances in medicine and surgical procedures, many cardiologists approach blocked coronary arteries in much the way a mechanic approaches a blocked gas line in a car: "Gotta open it up, maybe tear it out and replace it." Gotta open it up? *Angioplasty.* Tear it out and replace it? *Bypass surgery.*

Blockages or narrowing in the coronary arteries are never good things, but neither should they automatically put you first in line for the operating suite. As far as your cardiologist is concerned, blood vessels are supposed to be wide open, and if they're not, they need to be fixed. If you have the skill and technology to fix the problem, why not? Right? Well … not always.

First, from a physiologic point of view, your heart is not like the muffler on your car. If an artery is clogged, the body creates new pathways to pump blood through the heart. Unlike your muffler, your body is an intelligent being that actually solves some problems *naturally*. As we age, our body changes and reflects natural wear and tear. By age 50, you probably will not look "perfect." Unfortunately, many Americans have the misguided understanding that everything should be perfect or fixed. But with your body, that's not always the case. Sometimes, trying to fix every problem—with the most sophisticated tools available—causes more harm than good.

Second, invasive therapy is not necessarily better than conservative management. In many instances, depending on your problem, conservative management may have better outcomes and far fewer side effects. This is particularly true for anyone over the age of 70. For older adults, the risk of developing complications after surgery is higher than in younger people.

In addition, in over 60% of cases where a patient presented with blocked arteries, heart attacks are caused by blockages in blood vessels that appeared normal during angiograms. They're not caused by the blood vessels that triggered all the concern in the first place. Combine that with the very high risks of developing infection after surgery and an equally high risk for sustaining irreversible cognitive declines, the case for invasive therapy should be carefully assessed.

Whenever you are faced with the challenge of choosing aggressive medical therapy over conservative management—whether it's heart disease or back pain—you must address these key questions:

- Will the recommended treatment prolong my life?

- Will it prevent me from having bigger problems later in life?

- Will it improve my quality of life and reduce any current symptoms?

- What data is available to show the benefits of an invasive therapy over a conservative one?

- What are the potential side effects and what is my risk of getting one?

There are thousands of examples of unnecessary surgeries and procedures and, as a geriatrician, I see the effects of inappropriate care every day. But rather than giving a story of shocking proportions and family disaster, I want to offer up a more nuanced, complex account of the effects of choosing more over less. Ultimately, the path is not always clear-cut, black or white. When it comes to your health, sometimes the situation is frustratingly grey—and, in treating an illness or disease, you have to weigh your options and address your risks.

Consider this man's story:

One of my patients, a remarkably healthy 78-year-old, used to vacation in Europe every year. To make sure everything was ticking along the way it should, he scheduled a treadmill stress test each time before he went out of town. Three years ago, for the first time, the results of the test were abnormal. In order to evaluate the situation, his doctor did an angiogram, a procedure where radioactive dye is injected into the coronary arteries in order to detect any blockages that may prevent adequate blood from reaching the heart. The results showed that three coronary arteries were severely narrowed and the next day, he underwent coronary bypass surgery.

Thankfully, the surgery went well. When I visited him a few weeks afterward, he couldn't quit praising the cardiologist and surgeon. "I was a walking time bomb," he kept saying. "Thank God they found it in time." He had not consulted me about the surgery and I was thankful that he seemed to be recovering fine. However, a year later, the picture wasn't so rosy. His heart never gave him any problems, but he had still not regained his physical strength. He used a walker, feared falling, and needed help with basic daily tasks. The biggest problem, which caught everyone in his family off-guard, was his severely deteriorating memory. He struggled to remember people's names or tasks he'd accomplished only minutes before.

Although he did not know this at the time of his surgery, profound memory loss is a well-recognized complication of bypass surgery. Doctors consider it an acceptable tradeoff for a presumably lifesaving procedure.

Despite all of his problems, he continued to praise his cardiologist—who most certainly had saved his life. But what kind of life did he leave him with? He would never travel again, he did not remember his grandchildren, and could not feed himself. As far as

I am concerned, the cardiologist did not save my patient's life, he ruined it.

Prior to his surgery, this elderly man was not only robust and vibrant, but presented with *zero* symptoms of heart disease. He never should have had the stress test in the first place. Almost certainly, the narrowed arteries had been that way for years. For patients like this, there is no evidence that surgery prolongs life or reduces the risk of heart attacks. Yes, surgery can reduce chest pain, breathlessness, or other symptoms, but this man had no symptoms!

For older adults, coronary bypass surgery comes along with a 40% change of cognitive impairment. So, for many people, this is where the issue becomes grayer. While I ardently believe that this man should never have received a stress test or undergone surgery, many physicians disagree with me. So, as the patient, you need to be aware of every possible approach and every possible outcome. Would you accept the risk of memory loss over the risk of a heart attack?

When to have open-heart surgery
If a physician recommends open-heart surgery, here is the current consensus of when it should be done.

- *If you have an angiogram and the cardiologists finds:*

  ○ *Blockage of the left main coronary artery – the "widow maker." Here surgery dramatically prolongs life.*
  ○ *If you have significant blockage of three or more vessels and you have other conditions to impair heart function.. This is measured as the percentage of blood pumped out of the heart with each contraction. This is called the "ejection fraction" and if less than 40% surgery may be warranted.*

- *If your doctor tells you that three or more vessels are blocked, he will almost always recommend surgery. But surgery only benefits if you refuse or unable to live a heart-healthy life. Even for 50-year-old adults, the average prolongation of life is only seven months.*

- *Over the age of 70 or 75, the only indication for any surgical intervention is to relieve symptoms that have not responded to medical management and interfere with your quality of life. There is no evidence that your life will be prolonged (more likely it will be shortened), the risk of a heart attack will not decrease and the complications including death and memory loss become unacceptably high.*

A doctor's greatest failure?

For any patient of any age, choosing to do less rather than more is often a very difficult decision. Sometimes the decisions can be extremely clear, other times more murky. But, take a moment to consider *why* we have such a propensity to do more. As American physicians, we are trained to do *anything* to avoid death. Death is a doctor's greatest failure. 90% of a patient's health care dollars are spent in the last 10% of his or her life. We will do anything and everything possible to prolong life, even when there is no evidence to support it. As patients and physicians, we cling to any chance of survival no matter how small. Perhaps this is at the core of why we prefer aggressive therapy over conservative management.

Ultimately, I come to this debate with a different point of view. As a geriatrician, it is my greatest privilege to help a patient die with dignity. Older adults have accepted the reality that death is inevitable and most of them do not want the extra therapy or medication that may prolong life. When facing terminal illness, adults of any age should seriously consider the benefits and side effects of every medical therapy. Sometimes less is more.

Consider these cases:

A few years ago I had the privilege of treating two men, both in their 70s, who were diagnosed with inoperable lung cancer. Their x-rays looked very similar and they had the same features on biopsy. Interestingly, neither patient had any major symptoms of lung cancer. They had not lost weight, did not have a significant cough, and had not had a recent infection. Although these two patients had the exact same condition, they approached their therapy in two distinctly different ways.

One patient was immediately treated with intensive radiotherapy. The aggressive treatment was extremely hard on his body and his health progressively deteriorated. He became ill, developed an infection, and totally lost his appetite. Despite significant attempts at rehabilitation, he become progressively weaker and died within three months of the diagnosis.

The other patient was recommended the same aggressive radiotherapy, but he came to see me before making any decision about his treatment. He asked me this question: "Will radiotherapy prolong my life?" The answer was no. There was no evidence that it would either cure him or prolong his life. It could relieve symptoms, but he did not have any. In addition, we could not predict how quickly the tumor would grow. It could grow extremely rapidly or it could grow very slowly. We could not predict how long he would remain symptom-free. In the end, he elected to have no therapy at all. We just observed him and kept any discomfort at bay. Incredibly, he had three wonderful years before he died, not from the tumor but from a massive stroke.

The moral of these two men's stories is that you have to **weigh your risk**. When the evidence is questionable and the outcomes unclear, I will lay my bets with doing less instead of more. In the end, your greatest assess it quality of life, not quantity.

Don't blindly trust *any* doctor – myself included!

I hope after reading these stories and learning of the consequences of being a disempowered patient, you can approach your own care with a greater degree of empowerment. However, remember that no doctor is infallible—including me! Nothing that I have said is an ultimate truth. Your health care is rarely a black-and-white landscape. Sometimes you *do* need the best and newest treatment. Sometimes you need to exhaust every possible therapy to ensure success. Sometimes conservative management is not the best approach.

The message is simple: *you* are the best advocate for your health. *You* must assume the responsibility to understand your own illness. It is *your* responsibility to engage with the medical system early to detect disease and prevent illness. Ultimately, *you* have the right to make decisions about every course of action a physician recommends. Be passionate about your own health!

CHAPTER 11
DO IT *YOUR* WAY

So, that's it: nine steps to live a healthier, happier, more passionate life.

> *Passion. Peace. Love. Faith. Self-love. Sex. Food. Exercise. Empowerment.*

Each of these steps work together, one building on the other to help you find your own approach to lifelong health. But none of it is sustainable without one, final step to consider: **Do it *your* way.** Health is a journey: an ever-evolving path where we make choices each day to do the right thing. But those choices change. What's right for me may not be right for you. What's healthy today may be unhealthy tomorrow.

There is no one definitive way to live *your* life well. Each step in this Longevity plan is merely a guide, a framework for you to use in your own situation. I have not given you a specific prayer to pray, nor have I supplied a detailed diet to follow. I avoid those sort of specific guidelines for a reason! You have to *decide* what works. You are responsible for creating the details of *your* Longevity plan.

Health is, far too often, too prescriptive, too limiting, and too structured. If you can determine the details of what it takes to live a healthier, happier life, then your chances of success are much greater than any specific recipe someone else could give you. This is especially true as you age, because living a healthy life at 35 is different than at 65. It's time to abandon the stereotypes associated with health. Health is not limited to the super-skinny, the super-fit, or the super-peaceful. In fact, abandon the idea of extremes altogether. The road to lifelong health is not a narrow one.

The final step in Dr. David's Longevity plan is to have *more* freedom to live your healthy, happy and independent life. You decide what works, what doesn't, and what kind of life you want to lead—at every age. You have the freedom to create your own path for lifelong health.

What to choose, now?

Every seven seconds another baby boomer turns 60. That's an astounding statistic! Even more astounding: no one is ready for us. Politicians are scrambling to protect Social Security and Medicare. The corporate world fears the mounting pensions and the dwindling work force. Communities certainly aren't prepared, with poor public transportation and limited opportunities for social engagement. And as quality primary care grows increasingly scarce, I think it's clear that doctors and hospitals aren't prepared. But more than any social, political, and economic consideration, the biggest question is: Are *you* prepared? For most of us, I fear the answer is no.

Let me share my story.

A few years ago my daughter graduated from college. She moved home, found a job, bought a house, and embarked on the very arduous task of finding herself … of defining who she was without the context of school or parents. We were talking the other day and she said to me, "Dad, I had no idea it would be this tough! No one prepared me for this quarter-life crisis!" A quarter-life crisis—can you believe it? At 25, she has the world ahead of her! And yet she feels like she's struggling to find her place. With a little reflection, though, I understood her completely, because we were both facing new phases of life. She and I were in the very same situation. Whether I wanted to admit it or not, I too was struggling to find my place in this new phase of life. If she was facing a quarter-life crisis, I was facing a three-quarter-life crisis. It wasn't the typical midlife crisis often portrayed on TV (I didn't go out and buy a Harley, nor did I dye my hair and inject myself with Botox). I don't want to be younger. In fact, I'm happy those days are behind me. Rather, I want to define myself in this next phase of life. It's not about going back; it's about moving forward.

But just like my 25-year-old daughter, I have hopes and dreams, fears and worries.

Life at 65 is a whole new world. My children are grown, my mortgage is almost paid, the days of college tuition are almost over, and everything seems to be changing. For the first time in decades, this chapter is about *me*, not about my job, my kids, or my parents. I'm comfortable with myself, past the insecurities of younger years, and—after 30 years of marriage—my wife and I know each other well. This new chapter in life offers a wealth of opportunities. I will finally have the time to try a new challenge and explore new areas to grow. It's my chance to give back to my community. I can be a better husband and a better parent. I can dote all over my grandchildren! I can travel more and start a new hobby. I'm finally free to do whatever I want, right?

All the opportunity and excitement also brings anxiety and concern. Will it all be downhill from here? What does that mean, anyway? Should I retire? If so, what will I do? Can I even *afford* to retire? How will I take care of my aging parents? Can I still take care of my children when they need me? How will I be a good grandparent? What will it take for me to age in place? How do I stay healthy? Do I really want to be so free?

So, just like my daughter, I have to face both sides of the equation—the good and the bad. Who will I be after 65? Will I fulfill the stereotypes, or defy them? Will I dwindle away and sit on the sidelines? Or will these really be the "golden years"? What kind of legacy will I leave?

Get prepared: 5 Questions Every Baby Boomer Must Ask

My story is not unique and the questions I have to face are universal. We must all get prepared for a new phase in life. In order to do so, you must ask some serious questions. How do you define yourself? How and where do you want to live? What do you want to do? What kind of legacy do you want to leave? How do you want to feel at 85?

You must make an active decision about your path. You cannot afford to be passive.

Question 1: How do you define yourself?

Baby boomers have been redefining traditional roles and stereotypes for decades. In fact, for baby boomers, the tendency to break the mold is a stereotype unto itself. Sociologists are already predicting how baby boomers will redefine "old age" and reinvent retirement.

To see glimpses of this, just look at the evolution of AARP, an organization that has certainly redefined itself in the last decade. *AARP Magazine* (a much preferable name to *Modern Maturity*) has the largest circulation in the world. But you won't find wrinkly old ladies on the cover … instead, you'll see Mick Jagger or Bo Derek! The images and expectations of older adults are changing before our eyes. William D Novelli, executive director of AARP, once said, "If you're looking for older Americans today—men and women 50 or older—don't look in a rocking chair and don't even look around the old fishing hole. You're much more likely to find people like these on Rollerblades or the Internet: they are inline and online— and mainline. Older people are not sitting off at the margins of our society … They are active, curious, and savvy. They have high expectations in life."

I definitely don't consider myself on the margins of society. I refuse to be sequestered off into some remote region while wait- ing to die! I am not just a spectator; I want to be part of the action. Without doubt, I certainly don't envision myself in a rocking chair crocheting afghans or in a nursing homes playing bingo.

So, the question is, how do you envision yourself? Before you begin the process of preparing for this next phase of life, consider this underlying requirement: **You must have the courage to break the mold.** Pave your own way and create your own defini- tion of how to keep yourself healthy, happy, and fulfilled. If you are going to be passionate about life and live each day to the fullest, you simply must abandon any idea of what you're supposed to be. Ultimately, that's the point! There is no definition of what you're supposed to be at 65 or 75 or 95 … only *you* can create it.

Question 2: How and where do you want to live?
Though seemingly benign, this question is a major one. After a certain age, we're almost expected to change the way we live. We're supposed to downsize—ease off the gas and start slowing. We're supposed to move to temperate climates and join the ranks of the

relaxed retirees. Right? But what if you don't want to slow down? What if you want to speed up? What if you want to stay in your hometown? Do you want to be only surrounded by people your age? Start asking yourself these questions now.

As an empty-nester myself, these questions about living aren't just the philosophical questions about speeding up or slowing down, but also real logistical questions about aging in place. For the first time in 26 years my wife and I live alone. Last year, our youngest son moved away to college and it was far more challenging than ever before. We are no longer raising children: they're all grown and living their own lives. Suddenly the focus of my days has shifted away from the kids—and on to us! In the last five years, we have gone from requesting a table of five to settling for a table for two.

Over five short years, our four-bedroom, two-story house went from full and bustling to quiet and empty. It's too big. Much to my surprise (and my children's dismay), we're actually thinking about selling it. I never though I'd want to leave the big house where my children grew up, but anything is possible. So now I have to ask myself ... where do I want to live? If I move now, I'll never want to move again. My living arrangement needs to accommodate my age; but what will that really take?

In the coming years, the issue of aging in place will become more and more prevalent. Every element of our day-to-day lives needs to accommodate every age and stage, from housing design to fitness equipment, cooking utensils, and public transportation. Instead of stairs leading up to the house, we should have ramps. Instead of stepping into a bathtub, a walk-in shower with a bench is probably more appropriate. Intercoms should be standard amenities and bathrooms should be easily accessible. Doors should be wide, gardens should be manageable and maintenance should be easy. But beyond architectural design, our communities should ease the aging process. Public transportation should be available, price of living should be manageable, and safety should be a priority. Unfortunately, in many cities, this may not be readily available. Without governmental and community intervention, aging in place may be difficult.

Concerns about logistics lead to the larger question of community. Does your community make it easy to live the way *you* want to live? Will it be easy for you to remain active and engaged? Will it be easy for you to remain healthy and independent?

For many people, retirement communities offer a wonderful solution. Designed with the needs of an older consumer in mind, the houses in these pre-planned areas are already elder-friendly. Everything is wheelchair-accessible, and pre-existing infrastructures are created to accommodate any needs that may arise such as laundry services, in-home nursing care, and transportation. Retirement communities can offer the best of all worlds: convenience, ease, and community. But what if you don't want to move? What if a retirement community is simply not for you? It's important we find alternatives within our own communities to support anyone who seeks to age in place.

Question 3: What do you want to do?

Again, this seemingly benign question has heavy undertones. We don't really expect our retirees to "do" anything. They retire from work and that's the end of it. Volunteering may be in the cards, or maybe some traveling, but other than that life should be pretty free. Right? Well, for many of us, reaching the age where there's "nothing to do" is terrifying.

To retire or not to retire:

For most of our lives, work *is* what we do. Work defines us and provides structure throughout the day. Work may not be fun or engaging, but it's a huge component of life. So in order to answer the question "What do you want to do," you may want to start with another question: "Do you want to retire?" or "What does it *mean* to retire?"

If you're like me, the classic sort of retirement is nowhere in sight. Work is my career *and* my avocation: it's a passion that I cannot imagine leaving. It is a very positive and healthy component of my life. However, just because I see no need to retire does not keep me from seeking change and growth in my current situation. For me, the changes at work are less about retirement and more about enjoyment. At 65, I'm able to seek out more opportunities to enjoy my work, as well as eliminate the less appealing aspects of working life. I don't need to look beyond my present situation to find the next fulfilling challenge.

My wife, on the other hand, represents another side of the retirement coin. She loves practicing medicine, but she'd like to scale back in the next several years and make room for other pursuits. In essence, she wants to have her cake and eat it, too! She wants to be "semi-retired." She plans to participate in medical missions or join Doctors Without Borders, helping people in developing countries gain access to quality medical care. She also intends to travel, garden, learn to speak Spanish, and explore new hobbies. Far from the traditional model of retiring to sunny Florida and playing tennis, Francie's idea of retirement suits her: it will keep her motivated and engaged throughout life. She'll still work and she'll have plenty "to do," but it will be in a completely new context with new challenges and obstacles.

For others, retirement is the perfect opportunity to build new dreams … or fulfill old ones. Take the story of Mrs. Jean Marotta, happily married for 46 years with three children and four grandchildren. At age 16, she abandoned her dream of becoming a nurse; at that time, it would have required that she live in the hospital to receive her training. Her father refused to let her live away from home, so she tucked her dream away, married at a young age, had a wonderful life as a homemaker and raised her children. But she never forgot her dream. In 1998, when her daughter had a baby, Jean finally confessed her lifelong wish to become a nurse. "Go to school now!" her daughter urged. That urging was all she needed, and Jean promptly entered nursing school. She describes the experience as follows:

That was the beginning of a three-year odyssey that ended in my graduation as a registered nurse from Maria College (in Albany New York) in May 2002. At the graduation ceremony, I won an award for the highest average in my class (3.9). Walking across the stage

I wanted to shout, "If I can do this, anyone can!" It was the most satisfying, wonderful, ecstatic experience of my life.

I loved everything about the learning process. I learned volumes about myself. I learned that I can do anything I set my mind to and can accomplish any goal. All one needs is determination, desire, interest, and love of what you're doing. I had lots of support from my husband, children, and grandchildren. They were my cheering section."

Today she works as a labor and delivery nurse and could not be happier. Jean wanted to finally *do* something that mattered to her. It wasn't about the job or the money; it was about finding a fulfilling path to follow.

For me, Francie, and Mrs. Marotta, retirement is a very personal issue. It is an opportunity to grow, evolve, and explore, both in and out of a traditional work setting.

Unfortunately, most of us misunderstand the issue of retirement. We tend to see it as a black-and-white issue: either you work or you don't. However, nothing is ever quite so black-and-white. This is especially true with the relationship between your work and your health. It's not so much about whether or not you *work*, but rather what you choose to do and how you feel about it. You should always work at something, whether it's for pay or not.

If you yearn to retire from the traditional work setting altogether, you must have a plan for post-retirement life. The main question is: **what challenge will you take on next?**

Eliminating the commitment and pressures of a career can offer you an opportunity to dive into new passionate pursuits; but you must be prepared. The classic example of the post-retirement work is the older volunteer. We have seen images of older adults volunteering throughout the decades, and there is an assumption that baby boomers will follow suit. Unfortunately, this may not be the case. In a recent report published by the Harvard School of Public Health, data indicates that baby boomers, unlike their parents, are significantly *less* involved. On average, boomers volunteer less, vote less, and are less likely to join community support groups.

These statistics seem to say that baby boomers are much more insulated and self-oriented than their "greatest generation" parents. So without a career to keep us motivated and involved, what does that mean for engagement in the next phase of life? I think the answer lies in redefining volunteerism for the boomer mentality. For me, volunteering must be more than walking dogs or licking envelopes. I want to contribute in a meaningful way; so every organization should be prepared to offer new, engaging avenues to give back. Harvard researchers summed it up perfectly: "…there is an opportunity to help boomers create a social legacy of profound importance. Their added years of life give them the chance. Their experiences in life give them the capability … and the need to come to terms with the world in a way that brings integrity to their life … Much may depend on the actions of the first wave of boomers, many of whom, while inspired in their formative years by President Kennedy's call to service, have been notably less involved in civic life than their parents … All of society will have a stake in the outcome."

Just as we broke barriers and defied expectations in the 1960s and 70s, we have the chance to do the same today. One can only hope that what you do—at any age—offers a vital and meaningful contribution to society. After retirement, the opportunities are endless. You may want to stay in your current career. Or you may want to start a new business, or switch careers. You may want to join the Peace Corps or become a full-time grandparent. You may want to run for office and help solve the many challenges our country must face. Whatever you choose to do must be a reflection of your own goals, desires, and passion.

You must choose to do *something*. Plan for the ideal situation and create an environment that's healthy for you. You may want to retire from work, but you must never retire from life. Keep working in any capacity that you like. By doing so, your health and your work go hand-in-hand. At this age, anything less simply isn't worth the effort.

Question 4: What legacy will you leave?

In many cultures around the world, elders are seen as sages and leaders, people to look up to and seek advice from, not to be relegated to a remote corner of society. As you age, the yearning to share life's lessons often grows strong. For me, the three-quarter-life crisis brought serious questions about my legacy. What am I doing here? What role have I played? Have I given back? What will I leave for those behind me? If these questions resonate with you, you're not alone. In the coming years, millions of baby boomers will shift their focus inward and find new ways to leave a positive legacy for generations to come.

A few years ago, I began to think seriously about my legacy. My father-in-law, Jim, was turning 87 and my daughter decided to capture his oral history through video. Over the course of three days, she videotaped her grandfather, asking him questions about his life, his thoughts, and his experiences. She learned things that even her mother did not know. Two years later, and just before his 89th birthday, he passed away. Today, my children have a permanent archive of their grandfather: a lasting reminder of who he was, and what he stood for. When we were watching Jim's video, I wondered what I will leave for my children and grandchildren. What will I leave for my community? What will I leave for the world?

Leaving a legacy is a personal process that only you can define. After 50 or 60 or 75 years on this earth, you have many life experiences to share and much wisdom to impart. Leaving a legacy may be on a small scale or a large one: from my father-in-law recording his memoirs, to Al Gore lobbying for recognition of global warming. Remember, the more you give, the greater your legacy will be. Coincidentally, the more you give, the healthier you will be.

It's time to ask yourself: What lessons can you teach those around you? What advice can you give about love or life or family? Who can you inspire? As baby boomers, we must reinvent the Elder Sages of American life, because we simply have too much to share.

Question 5: How do you want to feel at 85?

As you age, your feelings, emotions, and ideas will grow and evolve. You will challenge yourself to redefine what it means to "be old" - I guarantee it. We all feel young at heart. So, what *does* it mean to be old? What does it mean to "*feel*" old? Do you uphold the stereotype or do you break it? The answers come from within. But, you must ask yourself: how do you want to feel at 85? Do you want to feel engaged and inspired and active? Peaceful and reflective? Choose any adjective and make steps today to achieve it. *Start today* to be healthy and happy tomorrow.

Health is a huge component of successful aging; but health is more than an apple a day or a trip to the doctor. Every other element of your life, and every other question leading up to this one, contributes to your health. If you choose to take on life with zeal and passion, your body will follow. Your eyes will twinkle and your smile will convey a youthfulness that your children will envy. Things that mattered years ago may seem unimportant now. Things that seem important now will be gone in a few years. Your heart will open to the joys of everyday life, because life is precious and not to be taken for granted. Whether you consciously choose to do this or not, at some point there is a subconscious, natural shift in our thinking. With more years behind us than in front, your heart will open on its own.

Listen to your heart and the details of *your* Longevity plan will be obvious. Love more and be more faithful. Be kind to yourself and others. Put life in perspective and seek peace in every moment. Treat your body kindly, and it will return the favor. Life will still have ups and downs. There will be happiness and sadness, grief and joy, losses and gains. There will be love lost and love found, divorces and marriages, christenings and Bar Mitzvahs, sickness and health, successes and failures. Age is just a number; life does not stop at 65.

The bottom line is simple: *Carpe diem* … seize the day. Remain passionately involved, and life will be sweet.

APPENDIX
SECTION A: THE NEED TO KNOW GUIDE FOR SCREENING FOR DISEASE

SCREENING TESTS
Heart disease.
Tests performed depend on how many risk factors you have for heart disease. If you have more than three risk factors, more tests should be performed—and more frequently. The risk factors that increase your risk of disease are as follows:

- Over the age of 60
- More than one close relative who has had a heart attack, high blood pressure, or heart failure. The earlier the age of the attack, the higher the risk.
- Male
- Sedentary lifestyle
- Obesity
- High-fat diet
- High blood pressure
- Diabetes
- Anemia
- Chronic renal disease
- Elevated cholesterol
- Elevated homocysteine
- Elevated C reactive protein

The common tests that should be done include:

1. **Blood Pressure:** In addition to measuring your blood pressure, it is prudent to occasionally measure blood pressure at home or in the supermarket. Focus mainly in the top blood pressure and be concerned if the top or systolic value is ever above 135.

2. **EKG.** An EKG should be done at age 50 to obtain a baseline test. There is no evidence that an annual screening EKG to exclude coronary artery disease is of any value.

3. **Treadmill stress test.** This should only be considered in someone with three or more risk factors, and if normal should only be done again if symptoms suggestive of heart disease occur (chest pain, shortness of breath). There is no evidence that an annual treadmill stress test is of value in asymptomatic individuals.

4. **Cholesterol:** We now recognize this as such an important risk factor that an initial measurement at age 20 is recommended and every five years thereafter until age 50. Beyond age 50 the test should be done every two to three years. The important measurement are the total, the good or HDL, the bad or LDL cholesterol and triglycerides.

5. **Homocysteine:** This is an amino acid that, if elevated, is associated with a high risk of heart disease. If it's normal there is not good evidence that it should be measured more than once. Thus, at the moment, every five years seems prudent.

6. **C reactive protein.** This test is a measure of inflammation. It should be measured at age 50 and in high-risk individuals every two to three years thereafter.

7. **Hemoglobin.** This is a screening test for anemia. In asymptomatic persons this test should be measured every two to three years until age 65 at which an annual test is routinely obtained.

8. **BUN and creatinine:** This test screens for kidney disease. It should be measured at age 50 and every three to five years in asymptomatic persons. An annual measurement

is warranted in persons with high blood pressure, diabetes or a history of cardiac or vascular disease or if you are over the age of 65.

9. **Blood sugar:** A random blood sugar should be obtained at age 50 and every one to three years thereafter, depending on risk factors for diabetes.

* A CAT scan of the heart should *never* be done to screen for coronary artery disease.

Screening for vascular disease.

Although common screening is controversial, here are the current recommendations.

1. Medicare recommends a single screening for Abdominal Aortic Aneurysm using a non-invasive ultrasound on one occasion in the first six months after reaching age 65.

2. There is no evidence that screening for carotid artery disease is of value in asymptomatic individuals.

3. There is no evidence that screening for vascular disease is of value in asymptomatic individuals.

Screening for cancer

Breast cancer

Screening for breast cancer is much more controversial that most believe. There are problems with false positives (an abnormality that turns out not to be breast cancer) and false negatives (screening tests miss the cancer). Cost is also a concern. Here are some general guidelines:

1. Self-examinations. From age 20 onward, every women should be knowledgeable about breast self-examination.

Screening for lumps should be done three or four times a year.

2. Breast exam by a health care provider should be done annually.

3. Mammograms should be done for the first time at age 50. There is little evidence that an annual examination is warranted in someone who is at low risk of breast cancer and in whom the mammogram is normal. Most are done annually. Every two to three years may well be adequate. Mammograms should continue in everyone with a productive life expectancy of 10 years or more. Beyond age 75 the frequency of mammograms remains controversial.

4. Mammograms should be done earlier and more frequently in women at high risk of breast cancer. This includes:
    a. The first mammogram should be done at age 40 in anyone who has had one or more close relatives with the diagnosis. The younger the age at diagnosis the more important it is to begin screening at a young age. Thereafter an annual mammogram should be done.

    b. Annual mammograms should be done in anyone who has had an abnormality identified on a previous mammogram.

Colon cancer

Screening for colon cancer is critically important as it is the second most common cancer in men and women, occurring almost as frequently in women as breast cancer. Screening includes:

1. An annual examination of the stool for microscopic amounts of blood. Although not pleasant, it can be done at home using cards. Today home tests are also available.

2. In low-risk individuals a colonoscopy should be done at age 50 and every five to 10 years thereafter.

3. Anyone who has a strong family history of colon cancer should consider a colonoscopy at an earlier age, particularly if the cancer has occurred under the age 50. There also some conditions that increase the risk of colon cancer, such as ulcerative colitis.

4. Your gastroenterologist may recommend earlier repeat colonoscopies if polyps or any other problem was identified.

Cervical cancer

The screening approach recommended by the American College of Obstetrics and Gynecology appears to offer the best advice to women. It recommends:

1. The first screening for cervical cancer includes a pelvic exam, and a PAP smear should be done three years after first intercourse or at age 21, whichever comes first.

2. Women up to age 30 should have an annual pelvic and PAP smear.

3. Women over the age of 30 may only need a pelvic and PAP smear every two to three years if three consecutive PAP smears were negative.

4. The college does recommend that in addition to a PAP smear women should also consider a Food and Drug Administration (FDA) approved test for the most dangerous forms of the human papilloma virus (HPV). If both tests are negative screening should only be performed every three years.

5. PAP smears are not needed for any woman who has had a hysterectomy with complete removal of the cervix for any benign reason.

6. PAP smear should be done annually on women who have had a hysterectomy because of abnormal cells. PAP smears can be discontinued if three annual tests show no abnormalities.

7. Provided three normal PAP smears have been obtained, further screening is not needed after the age of 70.

Lung cancer

Unfortunately there is no good screening test for early detection of lung cancer. The only practical current approach is a chest x-ray, but its value in early detection is minimal. At the current time, a special CT scan called a spiral or helical CT scan is being suggested as an approach to early detection. Its value, however, is not proven, too many small lesions are identified that turn out not to be cancerous and the amount of irradiation is excessively high. Large research programs are underway and in the near future new and better approaches to identifying lung cancer may be available.

Prostate cancer

This cancer is very common in men, and too few pay attention to screening for this disease. Unfortunately, there is still controversy about the value of screening, as there are many false positives, which lead to unnecessary biopsies and surgeries. There is no current evidence that annual screening affects the outcome of the disease. Although it's controversial, I believe that screening should be done; but patients must understand how to approach a positive test. Remember that the experts in the field believe that having this test is an individual decision and should only be done after fully understanding the potential benefits and possible harm. Here is my approach:

- A digital rectal examination must be done annually.

- PSA should be done after the risks and benefits have been discussed in detail and understood. In general I believe PSA is most valuable in men between the ages of 40 and 70. After that age the benefit is questionable, even though the risk of prostate cancer increases.

- Screening is more important in African Americans in whom the disease occurs earlier and is more aggressive, and in family members of men who have had prostate cancer.

- For many, the reassurance that the PSA will be normal is reason enough to get the PSA.

- If you have an elevated PSA:
    - If the PSA is found to moderately elevated, don't panic. Decide carefully if you want to have multiple biopsies.

    - Early detection of localized and asymptomatic prostate cancer has not been shown to be of any benefit.

    - Consider a watch-and-wait approach.

    - Repeat the PSA in six months. If it is unchanged do nothing and repeat in a year. If still unchanged repeat every year.

    - If the PSA has increased by 50% or more, go ahead and have the biopsy. In this circumstance your chances of identifying a cancer are higher.

Screening for Skin Cancer.

Everyone should be aware of the risks of skin cancer. Suntanning, exposure to the outdoors without sunscreen and sunburn are major risks factors for skin cancer. Skin cancer should be suspected if:

- A sore is present that does not heal.

- A mole that appears spontaneously or changes color. Particularly dangerous are moles on the palms of the hands, soles of the feet and genitalia.

- The American cancer society recommends skin cancer screening by a physicians every 3 years between the ages of 20 and 39 and annually thereafter.

Screening for osteoporosis

Every woman should have a bone density scan (DEXA scan) around the menopause and every five years thereafter to exclude osteoporosis. In some circumstances, more frequent testing may be needed in the years after the menopause to identify some women who lose excessive amount of bone during this time. Men develop osteoporosis too. Bone density may be warranted in older men (75 plus) who have lost an excessive amount of height or have an inexplicable fracture or bone pain that may be caused by osteoporosis. There are some who believe that every man should be screened for osteoporosis at aged 60 and every 5 years thereafter. However this approach is not yet proven.

Screening for diabetes

At the current time screening for diabetes is not recommended in healthy individuals. The American Diabetic Association recommends that anyone with the following risk factors should be screened:

- A family history of Type-1 or Type 2 diabetes

- A personal history of gestational diabetes that is diabetes diagnosed during pregnancy.

- Delivering a baby weighing more than nine pounds (diabetics often give birth to heavier babies)

- Obesity

- Being sedentary

- High blood pressure

- Being of African, Hispanic, Native American, or Pacific Island descent

The tests used to diagnose diabetes or increased risks of diabetes include:

- Fasting blood sugar. A level above 120 is considered to be abnormal.

- Glucose tolerance test, in which blood sugar is measured fasting and every 30 minutes after drinking 50 grams of glucose.

Additional screening tests

The following blood tests are often done every three to five years (unless otherwise stated) in those over the age of 65.

1. **A complete blood count (CBC).** This measures circulating red blood cells, white blood cells, and platelets. Its major function is to screen for anemia.

2. **Thyroid stimulating hormone (TSH).** This test measures thyroid function. Decreased thyroid function is very common in older persons.

3. **Serum calcium.** This test is often obtained, but is of limited value as a screening test. Measurement every two to three years is adequate.

4. **Vitamin B12.** Deficiency of vitamin B12 is very common in older persons. For this reason, this test should be obtained every three to five years (or more frequently if clinically indicated).

5. **Vitamin D.** We are now measuring Vitamin D levels in persons over age 75, particularly if they are largely housebound and spend little if any time outdoors. The test should be obtained every two to three years.

6. **Urine studies.** A simple test called a urinalysis should be done annually. It identifies protein in the urine (a sign of kidney disease) and blood sugar (diabetes). Other measurements are obtained, but the urinalysis offers little data as a screening test.

SECTION B: THE ANNUAL PHYSICAL

The physical examination

Test	Normal	Abnormal	What to do if abnormal
Pulse	70/min and regular	Very slow, fast or irregular	EKG
Blood Pressure	BP 120/80	Elevated: Systolic > 135 Diastolic > 90	Measure BP at home. Treat if systolic or diastolic consistently increased.
Blood Pressure in both arms	Equal in both arms	BP increased 15mm or more in 1 arm	Indicates narrowing of an artery. Always take BP in the arm with highest level
Blood pressure sitting and standing	No drop with standing	BP drops 15 mm or more with standing	May explain dizziness. May determine how high BP is treated.
Eyes	Normal color	May identify: 1. Jaundice 2. Anemia 3. Irregular pupil 4. Visual defects 5. Problems with eye movement	Order blood tests. If problems with movement or vision a complete neurological exam and perhaps referral to a specialist may be warranted
Ears.	Normal hearing, no wax, ear drum normal.	May identify: 1. Excessive wax 2. Fluid on the ear drum 3. loss of hearing	May remove excessive wax, refer for hearing test and treat for an ear problem if symptoms suggest it

Mouth	Normal teeth, no lesions, normal tonsils and throat	May identify; 1. Teeth or gum problems 2. Abnormal lesions in the mouth	May urge that you see a dentist, abnormal lesions may require further work up
Neck	No abnormalities.	May identify: 1. Enlarged lymph nodes 2. Enlarged salivary glands 3. Enlarged Thyroid	May require additional blood tests or scans to evaluate enlarged lymph nodes or thyroid
Carotid arteries	Easily felt	May identify: 1. Reduced or absent carotid pulse 2. A bruit (turbulence due to narrowing) when listening with a stethoscope	May order carotid Doppler's to exclude excessive narrowing of the carotid arteries. (This may only be required if there as symptoms suggesting mini strokes or other neurological problems.
Breasts	Normal	May identify: 1. Breast lump 2. Nipple discharge 3. Enlarged breast in a male (gynecomastia)	May order a mammogram. In a male with an enlarged breast, tests needed to identify the cause

Test	Normal	Abnormal	What to do if abnormal
Lungs	Normal breathing, no abnormalities when listening with a stethoscope (auscultation)	May identify 1. Mucus in large airways 2. Fluid in smallest lung pockets known as alveolae where oxygen is transferred into the body 3. Fluid in the sack surrounding the lung 4. Wheezing	Chest X Ray or CAT scan may be needed. Can diagnose chronic bronchitis, emphysema or asthma.
Simultaneous BP measurement in the arms and at the ankles	No enlargement Normal heart sounds	May identify 1. Enlarge left or right ventricle 2. Murmurs 3. Alterations of heart sounds 4. Heart irregularities	EKG and Echocardiogram may be needed. Depending on symptoms appropriate treatment instituted.
Abdomen	No pain, no masses (lump) no enlarged liver or spleen	May identify: 1. Abdominal pain 2. Enlarged liver or spleen 3. A mass in the abdomen 4. Enlarged kidneys 5. Enlarged Aorta – aortic aneurysm 6. Bruit on auscultation of the aorta or renal arteries	Depending on site of pain a stomach or bowel problem may be considered. Blood tests, ultrasound or CAT scans may be needed to evaluate other identified problems

Rectal Exam	Normal	May identify: 1. An enlarged prostate 2. A nodule in the prostate 3. A lump in the rectum 4. Hemorrhoids 5. Visible or microscopic blood in the stool	A PSA may be needed of prostate enlarged or a nodule noted. A colonoscopy should be considered of a lump or blood in the stool is identified.
Pelvic Examination	Normal	May identify: 1. Abnormalities on the vulva or external genitalia 2. Pain on examination 3. An abnormal cervix 4. Enlarged uterus 5. Enlarged ovaries	Will order a PAP smear and may refer to a gynecologist if a serious problem identified
Male Genitalia	Normal	May identify: 1. Abnormal lesions on the penis 2. Abnormal testicles	Additional tests may be needed. If a lump noted refer urologist.

Test	Normal	Abnormal	What to do if abnormal
Peripheral Vascular system	All pulses present and equal	May identify 1. Reduced or absent pulses in the lower limbs. 2. Bruit (turbulence on the femoral or popliteal [artery behind the knee] arteries 3. Changes in lower limbs suggesting peripheral vascular disease	Reduced pulses indicate great risk of heart attack and stroke. If symptoms warranted it, arterial studies may be needed. Excessive narrowing can be corrected by surgery.
Simultaneous BP measurement in the arms and at the ankles	BP in the leg equal to or higher than the arm.	May identify 1. BP in the leg 10% or more lower than in the arm.	A sensitive test of peripheral vascular disease. Most importantly indicates an 8 fold increase risk of heart attack and stroke.
Neurological system	Normal strength, no loss of sensation, normal reflexes and normal gait and balance	May identify: 1. Evidence of stroke 2. Abnormal sensation 3. Problems with gait and balance	May diagnose Parkinson's disease, stroke or peripheral neuropathy a common cause of pain. Referral to a neurologist may be needed.

Bones and Joints.	No pain on movement of joints no deformities. No spinal curvatures, no pain when examining back.	May identify: 1. Arthritis with either pain or deformities or both 2. Curvatures of the spine 3. Local pain when the back is examined.	Test or X rays needed to identify cause of arthritis or back pain. Local pain may aid with local pain therapy Osteoporosis suspected.
Nutritional evaluation	Normal weight, no evidence of nutritional deficiency	May identify: 1. Morbid obesity 2. Severe weight loss 3. Skin changes indicating nutritional deficiencies	Morbid obesity may warrant aggressive attempts at weight loss Being markedly underweight may be a clue to the presence of a cancer, severe infection or an inflammatory illness.
Skin	Normal color, no rashes, no suspicious lesions.	May identify: 1. Skin rashes 2. Excessive bruising 3. Suspicious lesions	Biopsy may be needed to identify cause of skin rash Common skin cancers are basal cell, squamous cell and melanoma.

SECTION C: GUIDELINES FOR COLON CANCER SCREENING

The American Cancer Center guidelines for screening of individuals at increased or high risk of developing colon cancer.

Cancer Risk	Age to begin Screening	Recommendation	Comments
INCREASED RISK			
A single small polyp identified on screening	3-6 years after removal of polyp	Colonoscopy	If the examination is normal, the patient can return to the normal guidelines.
A single large polyp or multiple polyps that have a high risk of malignancy	3 years after initial removal of the polyp	Colonoscopy	If normal repeat examination in three years. If normal then repeat exam every 5 years
Has had colorectal cancer	One year after surgery	Colonoscopy	If normal repeat examination in three years. If normal then repeat exam every 5 years
Colorectal cancer or a polyp in a close relative under the age of 60 or two or more relatives at any age	Age 40 or 10 years before the youngest age a relative was diagnosed with cancer	Colonoscopy	Every 5-10 years. Risk of cancer is only increased if the cancer has occurred in parents or sibling (first degree relatives). Risk is not increased if cancer was in uncles, aunts or cousins

VERY HIGH RISK			
Family history of familial polyposis a condition in which cancer almost always occurs	Puberty	Colonoscopy Suggest genetic testing	If genetic testing is positive a colectomy is warranted. Refer to a center specializing in this condition
Family history of hereditary non-polyposis colon cancer another condition in which cancer is very common	Age 21	Colonoscopy Suggest genetic testing	If the genetic test is positive or the patient has not had genetic testing perform colonoscopy every 2 years until age 40 and every year thereafter. Refer to a center specializing in this condition
Patient has either Ulcerative Colitis or Crohns disease, both of which have a high risk of cancer	Cancer risk increases 8 years after the onset of the disease if the entire colon is affected. Risk increased 12-15 years after the onset of the disease if only the left side of the colon is involved.	Colonoscopy	Every 1-2 years. Refer to a center specializing in these conditions

INDEX